'Herbs have always been the medicine of the people
– traditional remedies handed down from mo
to daughter or used by intuitive village heale

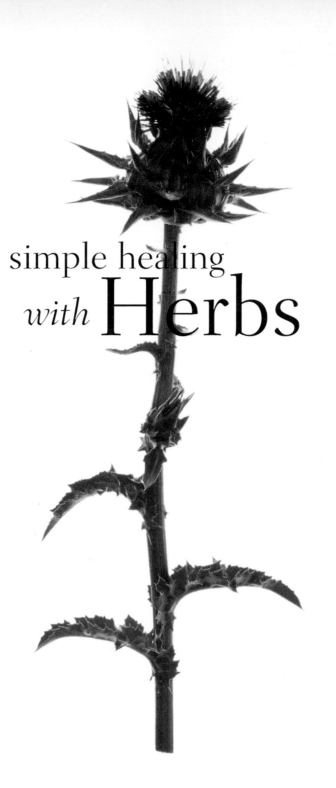

simple healing
with Herbs

Milk thistle *Silybum marianum*

Burdock *Arctium lappa*

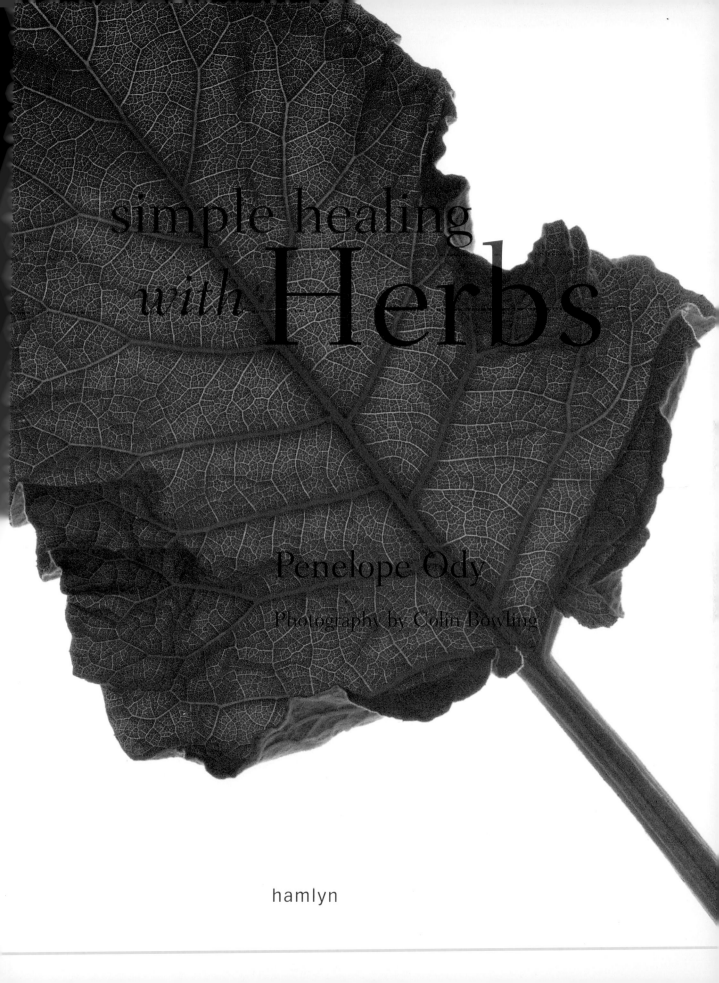

simple healing *with* Herbs

Penelope Ody

Photography by Colin Bowling

hamlyn

Publishing Director: Laura Bamford
Executive Editor: Jane McIntosh
Project Editor: Catharine Davey
Editor: Arlene Sobel
Assistant Editor: Nicola Hodgson
Creative Director: Keith Martin
Design Manager: Bryan Dunn
Executive Art Editor: Mark Stevens
Photography: Colin Bowling
Stylist: Sarah Cosgrove
Picture Researcher: Zoë Holtermann
Production Controller: Karina Han
Indexer: Hilary Bird

First published in Great Britain in 1999 by Hamlyn, a division of
Octopus Publishing Group Ltd, 2-4 Heron Quays
London E14 4JP

ISBN 0 600 59594 3

A CIP catalogue record of this book is available from the
British library

Typeset in Fairfield LH and 8½ on 13 pt Adobe Myriad

Printed in China

Contents

Warning

Herbal remedies should be used with care. Many herbs are unsuitable for use with particular medical conditions. Always refer to the safety warnings (*see pages* 7 and 116) before using any of the herbs. While the advice and information in this book are believed to be accurate, neither the author nor the publisher can accept any legal responsibility for any injury sustained whilst following any of the suggestions made herein.

How to use this book

This book is divided into five main sections beginning with a history of Herbal traditions (*see page* 8). This chapter traces the use of medicinal herbs from early beginnings in ancient Egypt and China through Galenic medicine to Medieval Europe and the New World.

The second section on Modern herbal medicine (*see page* 22) includes information on consulting a qualified herbalist and the wide range of over-the-counter remedies available today.

Self-help with herbs (*see page* 28) gives step-by-step advice on making basic herbal remedies in the home. With information on equipment and storage, this chapter provides easy-to-follow instructions on various basic procedures, including preparing infusions, decoctions, tinctures, and ointments.

Using herbs for health (*see page* 44) includes 120 commonly used medicinal herbs listed alphabetically by Latin name (*see page* 153 for an alphabetical index by common name). Each herb entry is illustrated with colour photography and lists information on which part of the plant is used, what medical actions are associated with each plant and which remedies are appropriate to each plant. The directory is cross referenced by a system of icons (see opposite for icon key) with the Ailments section (*see page* 86). The icons indicate which problem area each herb is most suited to treating. Cross referencing within the text indicates which herbs are directly referred to in the treatment options of the Ailments section.

Ailments – solving the problem (*see page* 86) is divided up by problem area into 12 sub sections. Each section suggests a variety of herbal treatment options for common problems and ailments. In addition, each section includes tip boxes, relating to the chapter as a whole, giving general advice on orthodox help, diet and supplements and preventative health. Thorough cross referencing throughout ensures that individual ailments can be related back to the relevant symptoms and causes.

Cautions are included, within both Using herbs for health and Ailments, stating which herbs have contraindications and suggesting when to seek orthodox and emergency help for particular ailments. A list of herbs with possible contraindications appears opposite, whilst herbs to avoid during pregnancy are listed in the Female reproductive section (*see page* 116). Refer to the chart in Babies and children for doses to suit children and the elderly (*see page* 152).

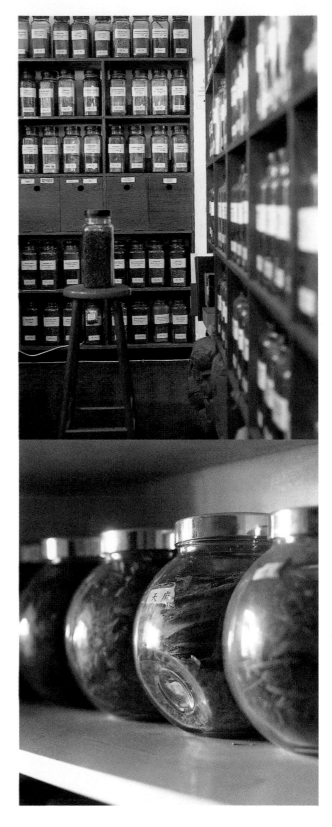

Using herbs correctly

While herbal medicine is generally regarded as quite safe, many of the plants involved are potentially toxic in high doses so need to be used with caution. Never exceed the stated dose and stop treatment if unexpected symptoms occur or existing ones worsen. Always be certain you are using the correct plant. This is especially important when collecting herbs in the wild: comfrey leaves are easily mistaken for foxglove, for example. Use a good wild plant key to identify specimens – and if in doubt, don't use it.

The right qualifications

In the United Kingdom, professional herbalists are members of either the National Institute of Medical Herbalists, using the initials MNIMH or FNIMH after their names, or The General Council and Register of Herbalists whose members use the initials MH. Both organizations offer comprehensive training for their members although they have a slightly different philosophical approach to herbalism: General Council members often tend more towards homeopathy, while Institute members may also be naturopaths and interested in diet.

Chinese medicine is covered by the Register of Traditional Chinese Medicine, whose members largely use a combination of acupuncture and Chinese herbs, while the newly formed College of Ayurveda ensures adequate standards for practitioners in this discipline.

Elsewhere in Europe there are French *phytotherapists* who are generally trained orthodox doctors who have studied plant medicine at post-graduate level; in Germany, alternative practitioners qualify as *heilpraktiker* and have comparable status with conventional GPs – these are also often keen herbalists who plant remedies for around two-thirds of their prescriptions.

Cautions to note:

The plants listed below may be contraindicated in certain circumstances. Cautions can be found in **Using herbs for health** (*see page* 44). Herbs to avoid during pregnancy can be found in **Female reproductive** (*see page* 116).

Aloe	**Elder**	**Myrrh**
Arnica	**Evening primrose**	**Nutmeg**
Basil	**Fennel**	**Parsley**
Bilberry	**Fenugreek**	**Passion flower**
Black cohosh	**Feverfew**	**Peppermint**
Bladderwrack	**Garlic**	**Raspberry**
Blue cohosh	**Ginger**	**Sage**
Borage	**Ginseng**	**Shepherd's purse**
Bugleweed	**Goat's rue**	**Siberian ginseng**
Cayenne	**Golden seal**	**St John's wort**
Celery	**Hemp agrimony**	**Thyme**
Chamomile	**Hops**	**White willow**
Chaste tree	**Hyssop**	**Wild yam**
Chinese angelica (*Dang Gui*)	**Ispaghula**	**Wood betony**
	Lady's mantle	**Wormwood**
Chinese rhubarb (*Da Huang*)	**Lavender**	**Yarrow**
	Liquorice	**Yellowdock**
Comfrey	**Meadowsweet**	**Valerian**
Cowslip	**Melilot**	**Vervain**
Devil's claw	**Motherwort**	

Ailment catagories for icons

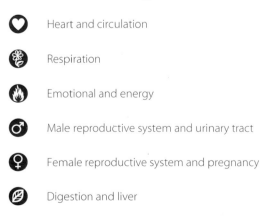

♥ Heart and circulation

❀ Respiration

🔥 Emotional and energy

♂ Male reproductive system and urinary tract

♀ Female reproductive system and pregnancy

🍃 Digestion and liver

  Infections

⚡ Aches and pains

👁 Eyes

💧 Glandular

  Skin and hair

  Children

Herbal
traditions

Herbs have been used in healing since the earliest times and are still the basis of some three-quarters of the world's medicines. Until the arrival of modern science there was little real understanding of why they act as they do, so the plants were often regarded as magical, while the traditional view of their actions – such as hot in the third degree – sounds very strange to modern Western ears.

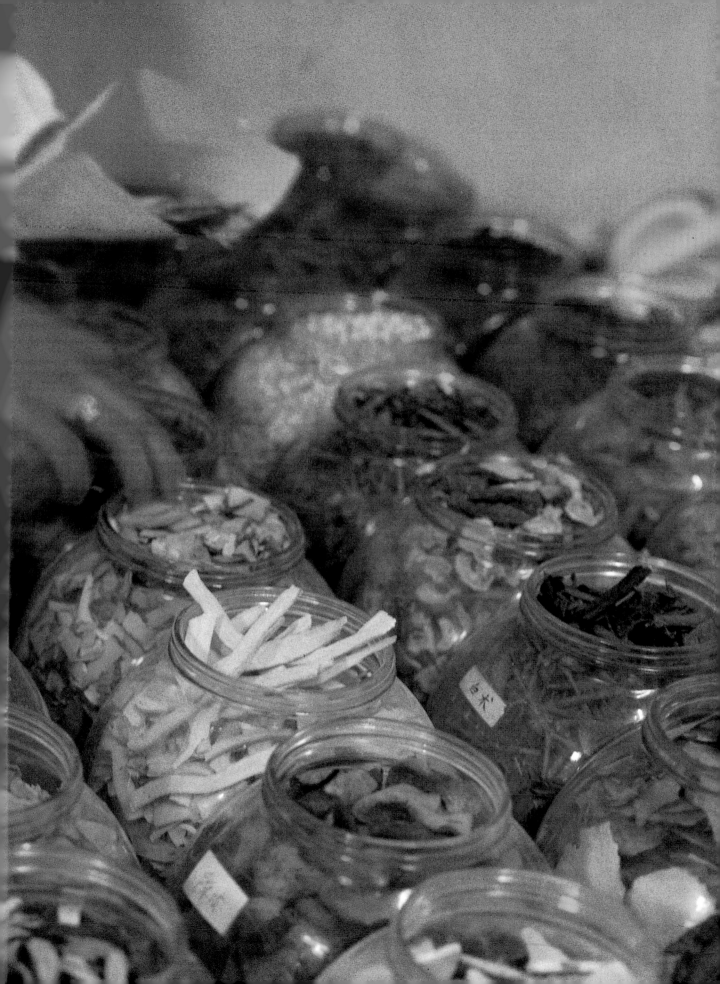

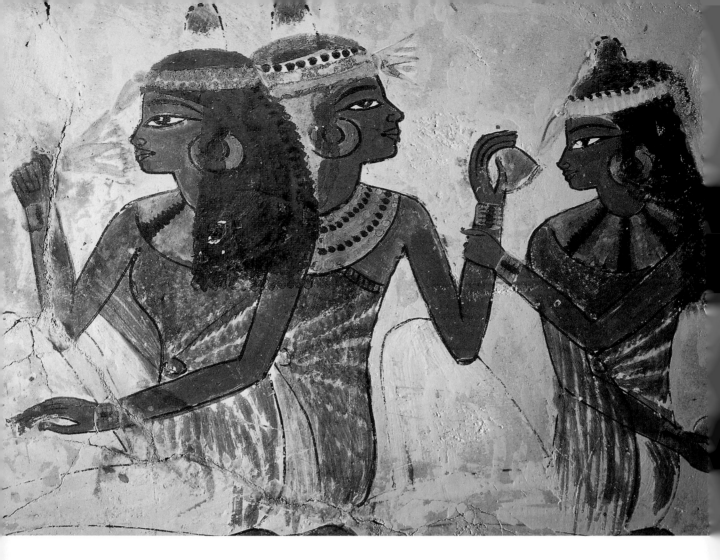

Rooted in history

Although in the West we have become used to shrink-wrapped pills and powerful synthetic drugs, herbs are still the only medicine available for as many as two-thirds of the world's people and are still the basis for many of modern medicine's most familiar drugs. Many of these herbs have been used for thousands of years.

Early beginnings

Plants have been valued and cultivated as medicines, as well as food, since the dawn of human civilization. Seeds from yarrow and marshmallow have been found among the grave goods in early Neanderthal burials, while traces of ephedra – a Chinese herb used in asthma treatments and the source of our modern drug, ephedrine – were found in Iraqi tombs dating back 60,000 years.

We can only guess at how these early people used their herbs, but they clearly valued them and supplied their dead with a sufficient quantity for the next world.

In the West our earliest surviving herbal manuscripts include Egyptian papyri dating from 1500BC, while Chinese herbal traditions derive from Shen Nong, a mythical emperor known as the 'divine husbandman' who introduced agriculture and is believed to have lived around 2000BC.

Many of the herbs listed in these surviving records are still used in very similar ways today: ancient Assyrians, for example, used astringent acacia (*Acacia nilotica*) leaves as a wound herb to stop bleeding, while chaste tree was prescribed for menstrual disorders – today we know that this herb has a potent effect on the female hormones. In the days of Rameses III (*c.* 1200BC) hemp (*Cannabis sativa*) was used for eye problems just as it may be prescribed for glaucoma today, while wormwood was not only recommended for intestinal parasites – as it is today – but also for 'pains of demonic origin'.

Early physicians were often priests and healing was as much a matter of pacifying evil spirits as prescribing curative brews. It is a connection still found in many traditional cultures even now, where the shaman or medicine man combines incantations, herbs, and trance states in an attempt to visit the spirit world and persuade whatever is troubling the patient to depart. These trances are often helped by hallucinogenic herbs, such as mescal buttons (*Lophophora williamsii*) taken by Mexican shamans or fly agaric (*Amanita muscaria*) used by Siberian healers.

In the West this close connection between religion, ritual, and remedies was commonplace until well beyond the Middle Ages: many old remedies combine prayer and ritual with a suitable herbal combination, while monastery physic gardens once formed the basis for primary health care.

Doctrine of Signatures

While modern science can now identify the particular chemicals in plants which contribute to their healing properties, our ancestors had to make do with trial and error. In China, Shen Nong, reputedly invented tea drinking when some leaves from a tea bush (*Camellia sinensis*) accidentally fell into a pot of water he was conveniently boiling underneath, and most cultures have a wealth of similar tales to explain other vital discoveries.

The identification of healing herbs was helped by the Doctrine of Signatures: a belief that the appearance of the plant provides clues to its therapeutic properties. Yellow-flowered herbs, for example, were believed to signify that the plant could be helpful for liver complaints since in jaundice the skin and the whites of the eyes become yellowish. The nodular roots of lesser celandine (*Ranunculus ficaria*) were similarly supposed to suggest haemorrhoids, and the plant is known as pilewort as a result. Many of these signatures do have some validity: dandelion and toadflax (*Linaria vulgaris*) – both yellow flowered – are good liver remedies; pilewort really will heal haemorrhoids.

Although the Doctrine is usually regarded in the West as a medieval belief or is sometimes attributed to Paracelsus (1493–1541) – a famous German physician and alchemist known as the 'father of chemistry', similar symbolic theories are found in

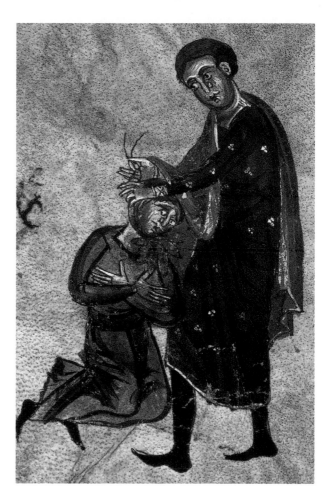

Opposite One of the earliest recorded use of herbs was in Egypt, where priests doubled as physicians. In this wall painting of a feast on the tomb of the priest Nahkt (c. 15th century BC) one woman passes another woman a mandrake root.

Above An Italian doctor treats his patient's headache with plantain root in this illustration from a medical treatise from the first half of the 13th century. Herbs like this one are still used as remedies today.

almost every traditional culture worldwide. The Chinese, for example, recommend bark from the trunk of the cinnamon tree (*Cinnamomum cassia*) as a warming remedy for chills and colds, but if the problem is chilblains on fingers or toes, then you need twigs from the ends of the cinnamon tree's branches to send the heat to the body's peripheries.

Following in Galen's footsteps

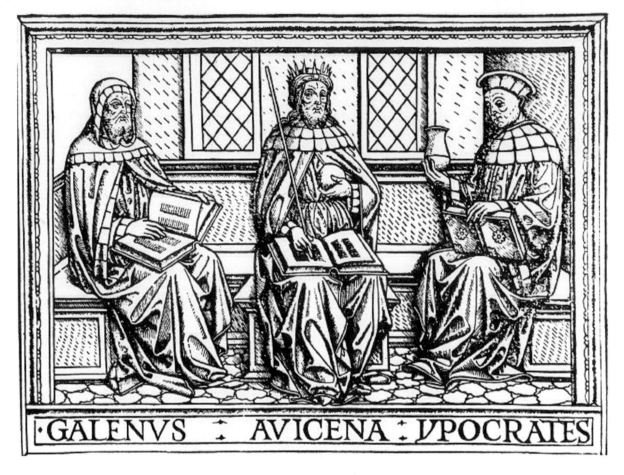

·GALENVS ⁘ AVICENA ⁘ VPOCRATES

Western herbalism has its roots in the medicine of the ancient Greeks and Romans, following traditions that date back to the days of Hippocrates in the 5th century BC. Both the use of herbs and the theories of health care followed by practitioners remained unchanged for 2000 years until the arrival of modern anatomy and physiology in the 17th century.

Greek medicine

Traditional Western medicine is often called Galenic medicine after Claudius Galenicus, known as Galen (*b*. 131AD), a Greek physician who spent almost all of his life in Rome. The Greeks believed that everything was made up of four elements – earth, air, fire and water. The nature of these elements influenced the seasons and all living things and they were also characterized by basic qualities – heat or cold, dryness or moisture. The elements also controlled the four vital bodily 'humors' and ancient doctors believed that human health depended on keeping these humors – blood, phlegm, yellow bile and black bile – in balance.

The humors were also believed to be largely responsible for human emotions and personalities. Depression and unhappiness, for example, were associated with the 'melancholic' temperament where black bile was dominant; to improve the mood it was thought necessary to 'purge' the black bile with remedies – such as senna pods (*Senna alexandrina*), figs, or liquorice – which today we would describe as strong laxatives.

Like the elements, the humors were also related to temperature and degree of dryness and could be balanced by herbs that had the opposite characteristics. Phlegm was, understandably, cold and damp, so herbs that were hot and dry – such as aniseed (*Pimpinella anisum*) and elder flowers – might be used to clear a productive cough or watery catarrh.

Arabic influences

After the fall of Rome in 410AD many of the original Greek texts were lost to Western Europe and survived only in the East – in Byzantium and, later, the Arab world. While much of Europe descended into the Dark Ages, Galenic theories were adopted and developed by generations of Arab scholars – perhaps most famously by Avicenna (*d.* 1037), whose *Canon of Medicine* travelled, via Moorish Spain, back to Western Europe and played a major role in re-establishing Galenic theories at early medical schools in Salerno and Montpellier. Welsh medical texts from the 13th century quote Avicenna extensively and his *Canon* continued to be used as a teaching text in some Italian universities until the 18th century.

Today these same Galenic traditions are at the heart of the Tibb or Unani medicine which is practised throughout the Moslem world. As with earlier Galenic practice, Tibb closely links lifestyle and personality to the humors and basic qualities, known today as *khawas*. Too much sleep, for example, is considered to increase dampness, while anger is thought to increase heating.

A wrong mix of activities and emotions thus creates *khawa* imbalance, which in turn upsets the humors and leads to ill health.

The spice and silk routes

While Arab scholars kept Galenic medicine alive, Arab merchants helped bring many new and exotic remedies to the West. European trade with India and China dates back to Roman times, but by the 9th century the Arabs controlled the spice routes and merchants could command high prices for such delicacies as nutmeg, cloves, or ginger.

These herbs were much valued by medieval herbalists. Hildegard of Bingen (1098–1179), a visionary German nun, wrote several books on health and healing as well a great deal of music. One of the herbs she used was galangal, which originates from China and Vietnam. Hildegard used the plant to treat heart complaints such as angina pectoris and it is still used in this way by German herbalists today. Hildegard's galangal would have travelled across Asia following the old silk route, and today we can find galangal roots among the fresh herbs in supermarkets.

Another common Eastern herb was turkey rhubarb, which also originated in China, where it is known as *Da Huang* or 'big yellow' from the distinctive colour of its roots and, as in the West, it has long been used for treating chronic constipation. The European name derives from the root's long journey through Asia Minor with the Arab traders and a mistaken early belief that the roots actually grew in Turkey.

Opposite Although they were separated by centuries, the triumvirate of Galen, Avicenna, and Hippocrates that is pictured here represents an unbroken line in the traditional herbal approach to Western medical treatment. In the 17th century, treatment was modernized as a result of scientific discoveries.

Right In this Persian illustration a king is being cauterized with herbs for leprosy. This was a rudimentary surgical procedure, compared to that of today.

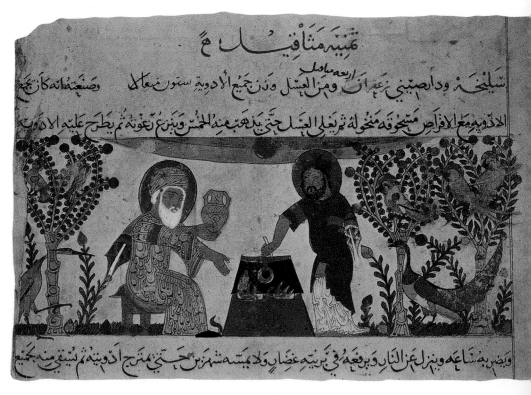

Steeped in myth and mystery

Herbs have always been the medicine of the people – traditional remedies handed down from mother to daughter or used by intuitive village healers. In earlier times their properties seemed magical and over the centuries healing plants have attracted their fair share of myths and legends.

Ancient echoes

For people who have no knowledge of biochemistry and pharmacology, the action of many herbs in healing disease could only be described in terms of magic. Causes of illness could not be subjected to modern scientific scrutiny but were often seen instead as invading evils. Traditional Chinese medicine still talks of the 'six evils' which can cause illness – wind, heat, cold, dryness, dampness, and 'summer heat' (not usually a problem in Northern Europe), while our Anglo-Saxon ancestors preferred to view illness in terms of 'elf-shot' and 'flying venoms'.

Herbs for treating these ailments, often those we would now describe as anti-inflammatory or antibacterial, were imbued with magical properties, and complex rites were necessary to maximize their potency.

Elecampane, now largely used for coughs and as a tonic after flu, was a favourite for elf-shot. In the *Leech Book of Bald*, written around the 9th century possibly by a physician who was working

Far left *In this 14th century painting of the Annunciation by the Italian artist Simone Martini the angel holds out a madonna lily to the Virgin Mary. The plant, once a pagan image, became a Christian symbol.*

Left *Herbal treatments and folk remedies were frequently associated with the magic of witchcraft, as evidenced by this 16th century Swedish illustration of fairies and elves on their nightly ritual dance.*

for Alfred the Great, sufferers are recommended to find their elecampane roots on 'Thursday evening when the sun is set' and were told to sing the 'Benedicite and Pater Noster' over the plant. Next morning the root could be safely dug up and, after more prayers and some time left lying under an altar, it was made into a tea and drunk.

Vestiges of these traditions have lingered into recent times in many areas, often giving rise to strange old wives remedies. My own grandmother always recommended wrapping one's left sock around the neck to treat a sore throat. She had no idea why – it was simply a folk remedy handed down for generations, and she always swore that it worked.

Witch's favourites

Perhaps because of their association with pre-Christian religions, many herbs even today have names linking them to witchcraft and ancient cults. Mullein is known as 'hag's taper', foxglove (*Digitalis purpurea*) was 'witch's gloves' and shepherd's purse 'witch's pouches'.

Some of these old pagan associations were translated into Christian orthodoxy: the Romans considered the madonna lily sacred to the goddess Juno and this symbolism was easily transferred to the Virgin Mary by the early Christians.

Others were not so lucky and became associated with fortune telling and evil mysteries. John Gerard, for example, who wrote his great herbal in 1597, cautioned that 'many olde odd wives fables are written of vervain tending to witchcraft and sorcery' and told his readers that he would not 'trouble their ears with such trifles'. Yet to the druids, vervain had been a holy plant, used in numerous rites and gathered at precise times depending on the

movement of the stars, while the Romans called it 'herb of grace', sacred to Jove, and gave it to messengers in wartime as surety for safe conduct. Today we use vervain for a wide range of nervous and digestive disorders, with or without any rituals attached.

Plants like deadly nightshade (*Atropa belladonna*), thornapple, and henbane (*Hyoscyamus niger*) have also been long associated with European witches. These plants are all hallucinogenic and witches are believed to have made a 'flying ointment' from the herbs which would be massaged into their skin to encourage trances or 'flying' – just as South American shamans still do today.

Surviving traditions

Even familiar hedgerow plants have their legends. The common elder tree was once known as nature's medicine chest since every part of it had some sort of therapeutic use: the bark and roots are strong purgatives – popular in the days when such treatment was central to balancing the humors, the leaves made a traditional 'green ointment' for bruises and minor wounds, the flowers eased chills, catarrh and fevers, while the fruit went into jams and wines, providing a good source of vitamins and minerals when fruit was scarce.

Small wonder, then, that the tree was regarded as magical: it was believed to be inhabited by the Elder Mother, or Hylde-Moer, whose permission was needed to cut the tree and take its healing branches – the obliging lady gave permission by staying quiet. In country districts until the 1930s it was still common to see elderly gentlemen doffing their hats to the tree, while it was considered bad luck to make a baby's cradle from elder wood in case the Hylde-Moer strangled the infant in revenge.

New ideas from the New World

Early settlers in America discovered a wealth of new healing plants to add to their traditional remedies brought from Europe. Many of these are now firm favourites with Old World herbalists, and there are new discoveries still emerging with plants like guarana and Peruvian cat's claw from South America joining the repertoire.

North American influence

The European settlers introduced some of their own favourite healing herbs, such as plantain, which became known as 'white man's foot' because it grew wherever the settlers penetrated, but they also absorbed a little of the North American Indian healing tradition. Herbs like boneset, echinacea, golden seal, Indian tobacco (*Lobelia inflata*), prickly ash (*Zanthoxylum americanum*), pleurisy root (*Asclepias tuberosa*) and American ginseng (*Panax quinquefolius*) were soon being added to traditional European recipes.

Native American medicine, like its modern day South American equivalent, was shamanistic, with the usual mix of ritual, spirit travelling, and herbal remedies, many of the latter being extremely complex. The Cherokee, for example, believed that rheumatism was caused by the vengeful spirits of slain deer so the shaman had to invoke the wolf and dog spirits, powerful enemies of the deer, to help him to cure the ailment; he also had around six hundred herbal formulas to choose from to help the spirits in their work.

For many Native American tribes, the healing process often involved lengthy periods in overheated 'sweat houses'. In the 1790s a New Hampshire herbalist, Samuel Thomson, incorporated this basic sweating technique into his *Improved System of Botanic Practice of Medicine* – a mixture of handbooks and patent nostrums which swept across America in the early years of the 19th century. By the 1830s he claimed three million active supporters. Central to Samuel Thomson's medical beliefs was the theory that 'all disease is caused by cold', which in the bitter New England winters may well have been accurate. His treatment included extensive use of diaphoretic (perspiration

inducing) herbs – such as cayenne and pepper – to encourage sweating, as well as plenty of steaming baths, which were intended to emulate the Indian sweat lodges.

In 1838, one of Thomson's followers, Dr Albert Isaiah Coffin, brought the new theory of 'botanic medicine' to Britain, with a similar mix of self-help books and patent nostrums. Largely because of the Industrial Revolution, the herbal folk medicine practised by generations of country dwellers had fallen from use and Coffin's system found an enthusiastic audience, especially among the urban poor of the newly industrialized towns. Extensive use of American herbs like Indian tobacco, cayenne, black cohosh and golden seal has characterized much of British herbal medicine ever since, and these herbs are used in many of our most traditional over-the-counter products. Such herbs are largely unknown in mainland Europe where the American 'botanic doctors' never ventured.

Some North American herbs have managed to cross the Channel, notably echinacea, which was extensively studied in Germany in the 1930s, and is now known as a potent antibacterial, antiviral and antifungal that is valuable in treating a wide range of infections.

Newcomers from the South

Exotic herbs from the Amazonian rain forests are also among the latest fashionable favourites to hit the health food shelves. Aphrodisiacs like catuaba (*Anemopaegma arvense*), tonics such as guarana (*Paullinia cupana*) , or 'cure-alls' like Peruvian cat's claw (*Uncaria tomentosa*) and paratudo (*Pfaffia paniculata*) are among the many now sold in assorted lozenges and extracts for regular, easy consumption.

The actions of these herbs are not always well understood and their Western use as over-the-counter prophylactics is often very different from traditional applications. Peruvian cat's claw, for example, is used by some Amazonian tribes as a contraceptive and by others as a remedy for rheumatism, gastric ulcers, dysentery and intestinal parasites. More recently researchers have used extracts of the plant for treating cancer, and so the herb tends to be marketed in the West as a tonic, immune stimulant and cancer preventative and is often taken in much higher doses than the original native extracts.

Many of these herbs are also collected from the wild, a process known as 'wild crafting', rather than grown in commercial cultivation. This practice is leading to severe shortages and long-term risk of extinction for many of the species involved. In North America golden seal, which is extremely difficult to cultivate, is already an endangered species, while the new demand for Peruvian cat's claw has led to extensive damage in the rain forests.

Left Native American medicine was shamanistic – based on ritual, spirits and herbs. In this 19th century illustration, the shaman wears a wolf skin and holds a tambourine in preparation for healing.

A hint of Eastern magic

The East has long had an important influence on Western herbal medicine. From ancient times, exotic spices have travelled along the spice and silk routes, while today both traditional Chinese medicine and Ayurveda are among the most popular of alternative health therapies.

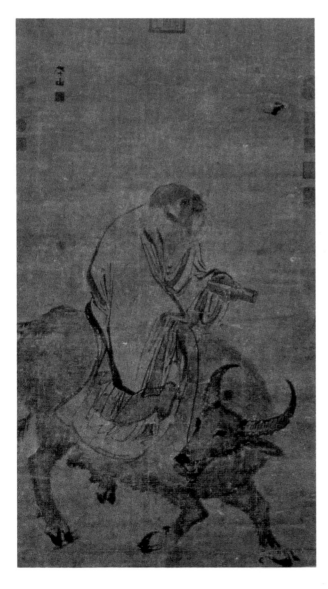

Balancing *Yin* and *Yang*

Like early Greek science, the traditional Chinese world view regarded everything as made up of basic elements: in this case there are five – earth, metal, water, wood, and fire – and, as with the Greek humors, these elements are also believed to control our bodily wellbeing and 'balance'.

The theory goes back at least 4000 years to the time of China's mythical Shen Nong, and the Yellow Emperor, Huang Ti, who is credited with the invention of medicine.

Just as the Western medicine of 2000BC was closely linked with religion, so too in China. Shen Nong and Huang Ti were Taoists and many early Chinese herbals and medicinal texts (such as the *Huang Ti Nei Ching Su Wên* or *Yellow Emperor's Canon of Internal Medicine*) are also rich in Taoist spiritual wisdom. Taoism is a way of life which concentrates on achieving prosperity, longevity, and even immortality through 'virtue' which, to its followers, means conformity to nature both within the individual and beyond. Herbs, especially potent tonics like reishi (a type of bracket fungus) were regarded as helping to strengthen this adherence to virtue and thus lead to a long life and good fortune.

Taoism also lays great store on opposites – beauty only exists because there is ugliness –thus giving rise to the theory of *Yin* and *Yang*, which is also important in traditional Chinese medicine. *Yang* and *Yin* are seen as two aspects of the whole – light and dark, male and female, hot and cold, and so on. These same forces affect human health and each of the five bodily organs of the five-element model which need to be kept in balance. Too much *Yang* and the organ is over stimulated, overheated, and prone to dryness; too much *Yin* and a cold, damp disease syndrome can result.

While Western traditions dating from the days of the Taoists have been gradually lost and eroded by changes in our culture and civilization, Chinese society has always preferred the *status quo* and change was not encouraged: 'may you live in interesting times' is a Chinese curse, not a blessing.

The result is an almost unbroken healing tradition which has been gradually expanded and embellished, but where the basic core principles, established more than 4000 years ago, are virtually unchanged. Not only are many Chinese herbs still used in exactly the same ways described by Shen Nong, but the diagnostic techniques also closely mirror the teachings of the Yellow Emperor.

Chinese prescriptions are equally formalized and students have to learn by heart thousands of standard recipes used for treating the various disease syndromes of traditional Chinese medicine, which are always defined in terms of *Yin*, *Yang*, or five-element imbalance.

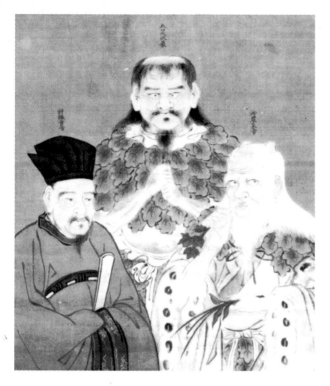

Far left The Taoist tradition, as exemplified by the great Chinese philosopher Lao–tzu (c. 604–531BC), here riding his ox, added a spiritual dimension to beliefs about health. Wellness was seen as a balance of Yin, Yang, and the five-elements, whereas illness was an imbalance, which needed to be treated with herbal remedies.

Left The Chinese equivalent of Hippocrates, Galen, and Avicenna are, as pictured on this scroll, the three legendary (and Taoist) emperors, Fu Hsi, Shen Nung, and Huang Ti, who are credited with inventing medicine. The Chinese still follow the techniques and treatments in texts such as the Yellow Emperor's Canon of Internal Medicine, written 4000 years ago.

Below This diagram, which shows the arrangements of pulses of the viscera and bowels, appeared in the early medical writings of the Han dynasty (200BC–220AD).

Ayurveda – a science of life

Indian traditional medicine is even older than traditional Chinese medicine and has its roots in health and hygiene theories that date back to the early Dravidian civilization of Southern India in around 5000BC. The earliest written text – the *Rig Veda* – is dated at around 2500BC.

The Indian word Ayurveda comes from *Ayur* meaning life and *Veda* which means knowledge, so Ayurveda is sometimes described as a 'knowledge of how to live', emphasizing that good health is the responsibility of the individual and not some pill-pushing practitioner. Like Galenic medicine, Ayurveda sees illness in terms of humoral imbalance, and although herbs play an important part in Ayurvedic treatments, diet and lifestyle are just as important. Therapy is likely to include an exercise regime, while diet can concentrate on tastes which, in Ayurvedic theory, need to be balanced and can have significant effects on wellbeing if they are not.

Many of the herbs used in India are well known in the West, although often the uses are rather different. We tend to classify basil as simply a pleasant flavouring for tomato or pasta dishes, while in India, basil (known as *tulsi*) is one of the most sacred herbs and has a powerful effect on our spiritual wellbeing. It is believed to clear the mind, strengthen faith and compassion, and increase the energies of love and devotion. Small wonder, then, that simply smelling that pot of basil on the kitchen windowsill makes us feel so good!

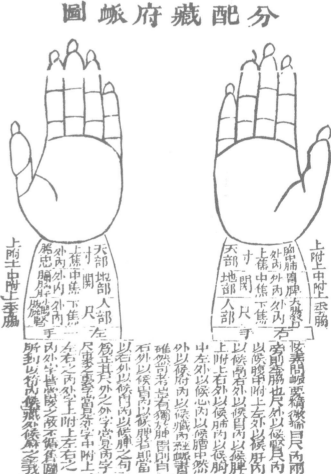

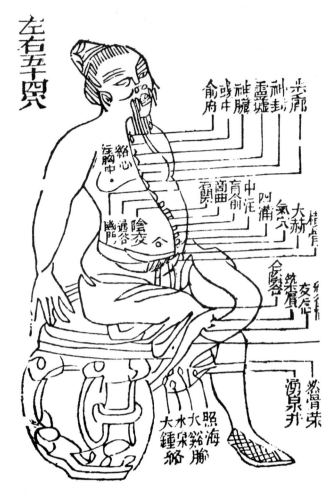

經腎陰少足
左右五十穴
俞或神靈神
府中膽墟封
絡心
渀胸
中
顧商中阿大
曲俞泣赫
幽通陰
門谷交
交
然容
谷
涌泉
大水水照
鍾宗谿海
絡腧

Balancing inner energies

Central to many traditional approaches to healing is the belief in some sort of vital force or energy which governs our health and wellbeing. To the Chinese it is Qi, in Ayurveda it is prana *and* agni, *while to the traditional Unani practitioner it is qawa. Whatever the name, all believe that maintaining the vigour of this inner energy is vital.*

Supporting the vital force

Modern orthodox medicine is 'allopathic', which means that treatment is by drugs which suppress symptoms; the popular alternative therapy, homeopathy, is based on a theory of combating symptoms by using remedies which would give you those same symptoms if you did not already have them. On one level, herbal medicine can be regarded as a type of allopathy, with tinctures and infusions used to counter obvious symptoms, but practitioners often prefer to talk in terms of 'restoring balance': using herbal remedies to strengthen the body's own healing powers to restore health.

This concept of an inner vital energy, which can be damaged by lifestyle and poor diet, is central to many of the traditional approaches to healing. Importantly, too, this vital energy does not exist purely in isolation, but is a reflection of the world around us.

In traditional Chinese medicine, this inner energy is *Qi* (or *ch'i*). *Qi* flows through the body in a network of channels which are familiar to us as acupuncture meridians, and the acupuncturist's needle is often intended to stimulate or control its flow. There are also many aspects to *Qi* – there is 'defence energy' used to combat invading evils, as well as the basic inherent *Qi* which we are born with and which is responsible for setting our own energy and creativity levels. These different aspects of *Qi* are focused on different parts of the body: the creative *Qi*, for example, resides largely in the kidneys, and symptoms of ageing are regarded in Chinese theory as a running down in this particular type of energy. Kidney *Qi* tonics like *He Shou Wu* are therefore a favourite remedy for a wide range of old-age symptoms – from prematurely greying hair to tinnitus and menopausal problems.

Chinese herbal tonics like ginseng, astragalus root, and liquorice are believed to generally strengthen and improve *Qi*.

Digestive fire

Ayurveda sees each individual as very much a part of the greater cosmos and views each as being influenced by the three primal forces: *prana* – the breath of life; *agni* – the spirit of light or fire; and *soma* – a manifestation of harmony, cohesiveness, and love. *Prana* is often equated with 'breath', and many yoga practices emphasize *pranayama* (breathing exercises), which are designed to support this inner force. More important for herbalists is the body's manifestation of *agni* as 'digestive fire'. *Agni* is responsible for absorbing and converting the nutrients we eat, destroying invading pathogens and toxins, and strengthening the immune system. It also converts the five elements of Ayurvedic theory – earth, water, fire, air, and ether (a nebulous nothingness that fills all space) – into humors which, like the Galenic humors, are believed to control our individual health and temperament.

If digestion were perfect, argues Ayurveda, there would be no humoral imbalance, but because it is not, imbalance and ill health can follow. So, most diseases are regarded as being caused by poor functioning of the digestive system; thus maintaining the vigour and strength of *agni* is central to treatment.

Food, drink, sensual gratification, light, fresh air and spiritual activities are all used to 'feed' the digestive fire and ensure that the correct mix of humors is produced.

Modern approaches

While the concepts of a vital inner force and a need for balance were familiar from Galenic medicine until well into the 17th century, the arrival of modern science soon began to erode the old beliefs. The French philosopher René Descartes (1596–1650) is generally credited with this new 'mechanist' approach which finally split science and medicine from religion. Factors which were not physically demonstrable – such as inner energy – were dismissed as mere acts of faith and relegated to the world of superstition and myth.

Traditional healers have, however, continued to focus on balancing inner energy, and the idea of a 'vital force' was central to Samuel Thomson's system of 'botanic medicine' in the 19th century (*see page* 17). His ideas continued to have a great influence on herbal medicine in Britain until well into the 1960s.

Today, many people are turning away from the mechanist approach and putting more emphasis on spirituality and man's place in the cosmos. The idea of an inner energy force is once more becoming a rational and acceptable concept and no longer one to dismiss, as Descartes and his generations of followers would have us believe.

Left Acupuncture, one of the primary forms of treatment in Chinese medicine, stimulates the Qi which runs along the meridian lines of the body. Here the kidney vessel of the lesser Yin is shown with 29 acupuncture spots.

Right One of the three primal forces of Ayurveda, agni, seen here, represents the spirit of light or fire. Herbalists view its role as 'digestive fire' as vital to the maintenance of good health.

Modern
herbal medicine

Today's herbal medicine is a combination of tradition and modern science. While research has been able to explain the actions of many healing plants others have remained a mystery, with unknown constituents still used in time-honoured fashion. Over-the-counter herbal remedies now offer a wide range of self-help medicines – a few are proven in clinical trials, but the majority simply use herbs as our ancestors have done for thousands of years.

CHAMOMILE ROMAN

CHAMOMILE ROMAN   10ml

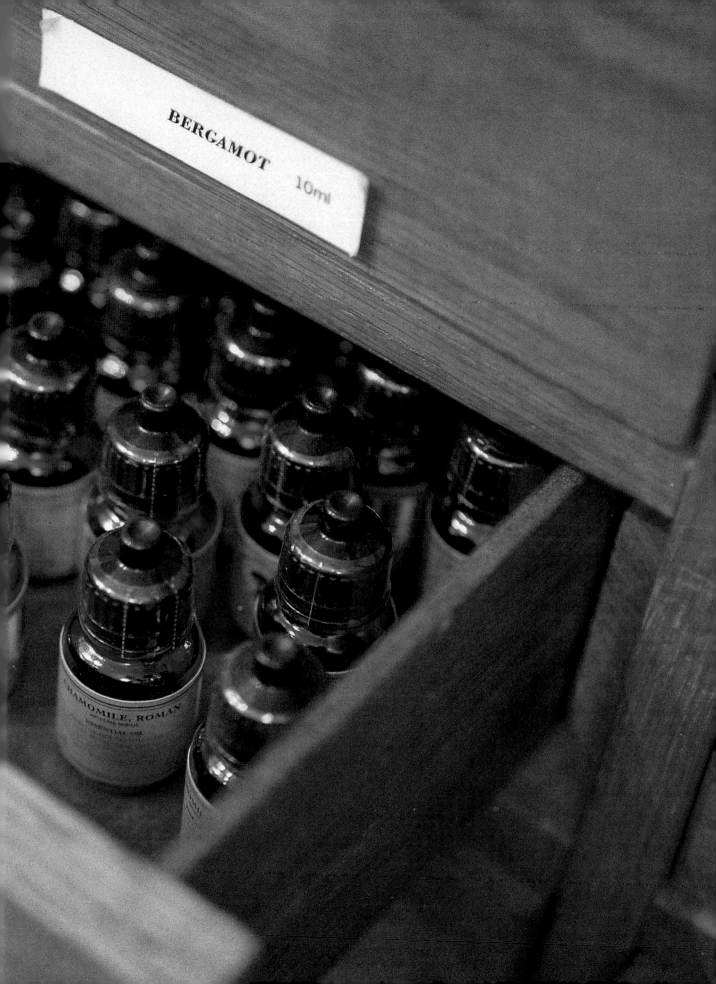

Herbal medicine today

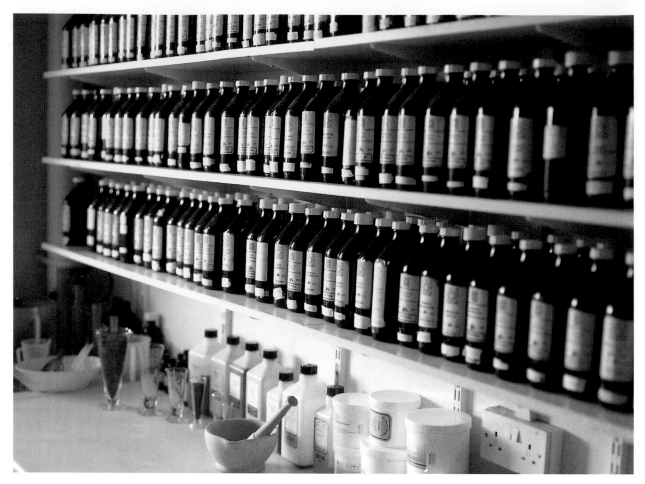

While many medical herbalists focus on restoring vital energy and take a holistic approach to healing, modern herbal medicine is also determinedly scientific and strictly regulated in many countries.

A balanced approach

Traditional herbalism has always been a holistic therapy – giving equal attention to body, mind and spirit. Herbs have been used in India for centuries to improve 'mental clarity' or compassion, while Chinese Taoists used herbs to increase mental and spiritual strength. Many professional practitioners in the West try to adopt a similar approach, using whole plants to heal the whole person. While many welcome a rigorous scientific analysis of herbal actions, others feel that the intuitive and spiritual side of herbal medicine is in danger of being lost and a satisfactory philosophy for modern herbal medicine has yet to be fully achieved.

Science has, however, continued to dominate the world of herbal medicine: not only do researchers continue to discover toxic plant constituents that can lead to over-enthusiastic bans of some potentially hazardous herbs, but also they are constantly presenting us with an array of new plant therapeutics. Plants like comfrey have been banned in many countries (comfrey contains carcinogenic alkaloids and has been shown to cause liver tumours in rats). Equally, the European herbalists of 70 years ago would have had little use for devil's claw, ginkgo, Peruvian cat's claw (*Uncaria tomentosa*), reishi mushrooms or even Siberian ginseng, but all of these are now regularly found on the shelves of health food stores.

Over-the-counter offerings

Herbal medicine is today a multi-million pound business – and it is still growing. Many people are looking to 'natural' medicines to replace the potent, synthesized drugs prescribed by orthodox practitioners. This may in part be due to concerns over side effects, although there is at the same time a preference for the less invasive and more intuitive approach of traditional herbalism.

The rules controlling the sale and dispensing of herbal medicines varies around the world. In some countries – such as Australia – everything must be licensed and tightly controlled, just as with pharmaceutical drugs. In others, as in Australia's neighbour New Zealand, there are virtually no rules or regulations and almost anything can be packaged and offered to the customer.

Use of various herbs is also restricted in different countries. In the United Kingdom potent plants such as lily of the valley (*Convallaria majalis*), which is used for heart disorders, or Samuel Thomson's favourite lobelia (*see page* 17), can only be prescribed by qualified practitioners. In parts of the United States, however, dried lobelia is sold by health food stores to all and sundry.

In some countries over-the-counter products can only make a claim to their efficacy if they are officially licensed, so that a pack of 'echinacea capsules' or 'marshmallow and peppermint tablets' can only be sold if the manufacturer gives no written recommendation on the package detailing what the products might actually be used to treat. This is obviously a disadvantage for the consumer as would-be buyers must depend on their own knowledge of herbs – or hope that the sales staff are suitably knowledgeable.

In Europe product licences are only granted where there is clear evidence of efficacy, which is usually allowed to take the form of research studies or information from official and herbal pharmacopoeias. Information must also be provided about the safety of the product, but once licensed the herbal products can be prescribed by doctors under national health insurance schemes.

Over the past few years, there have been moves to harmonize the rules and regulations controlling the use of herbal remedies throughout Europe, and there will soon be 'mutual recognition' of each country's licensed medicines. This will mean that herbal remedies with a full product licence manufactured in Germany or Italy, for example, will have that same status in the United Kingdom, and vice versa.

In the meantime there are plenty of European anomalies: St John's wort, for example, is licensed in Germany as an antidepressant and is a popular choice for orthodox prescriptions. In the United Kingdom, on the other hand, regulators believe that there is no tradition and little suitable scientific evidence for this action, so the producers are forced to market unlicensed St John's wort tablets as 'the sunshine remedy for dismal days', rather than as a respectable and effective antidepressant product.

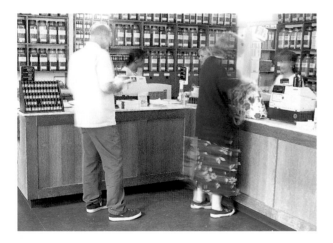

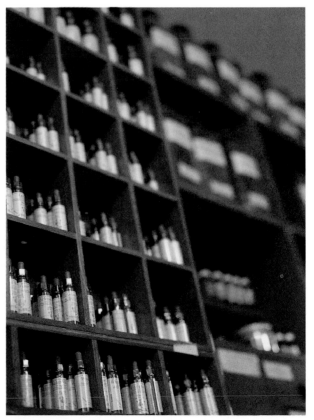

Opposite Concentrated extracts of herbs are made into remedies by medical herbalists in the well-stocked dispensary of this modern herbal medicine clinic in London. This particular clinic is located in a traditional hospital.

Above Dried herbs can be bought over-the-counter in larger health food shops, such as this shop in London.

Right Many health food shops sell essential oils and homeopathic remedies, as do many chemists.

Consulting a herbalist

While herbs can be ideal for self-help use at home, there are times when professional advice is needed. Fortunately there is a growing choice not only of qualified professional medical herbalists using Western herbs, but also of those trained in the related disciplines of Chinese herbal medicine and Ayurvedic medicine.

Visiting a practitioner

Herbalists treat a wide range of ailments, such as infections, aches and pains, menstrual disorders, high blood pressure, urinary dysfunction and digestive problems, as well as chronic conditions for which herbalism is often seen as a last resort – rheumatoid arthritis, chronic fatigue syndrome (ME) and asthma.

There is actually very little difference between consulting a practitioner and visiting a traditional doctor, except that the consultation will probably last 30 minutes or an hour instead of the more familiar 10 minutes. Indeed, many herbalists liken their approach to that of the old-fashioned family physician: they use careful listening and probing questions to uncover all of the relevant symptoms together with such conventional diagnostic techniques as feeling pulses, looking at tongues, testing urine and the classic clinical examinations of palpation, auscultation and percussion.

As well as reviewing the current illness, the herbalist will ask about medical history – previous health problems that may be contributing to the current imbalance, family tendencies and allergies, diet, lifestyle, stresses and worries.

At the end of the consultation, the patient does not simply leave with a prescription for the local pharmacist to dispense. In Britain, few pharmacies are willing to stock the hundreds of tinctures, creams, oils, powders, capsules or dried herbs that the medical herbalist needs to keep in stock, so all medical herbalists make and dispense their own remedies. Herbal medication is likely to be altered slightly after each consultation to reflect changes in the condition.

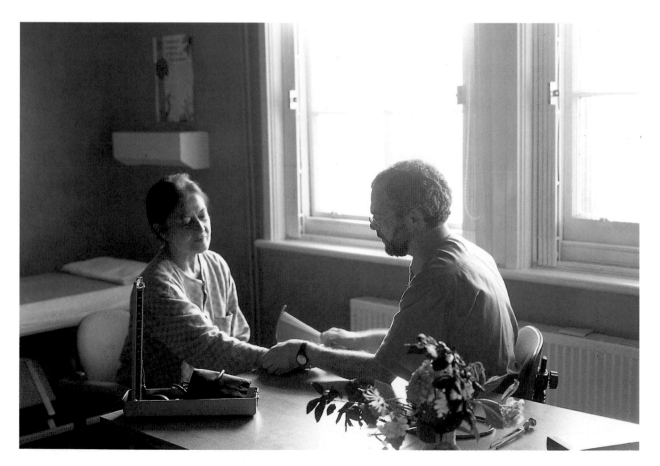

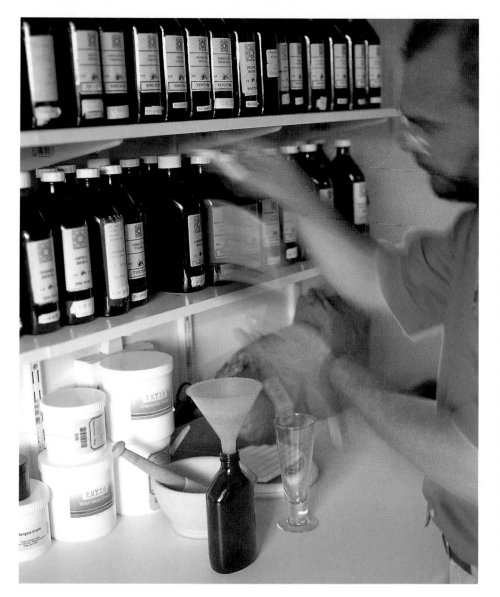

Opposite *This consultation, at a herbal medicine clinic in London, is similar to a traditonal consultation with a doctor, but longer lasting and more detailed. As well as discussing your medical history and symptoms, and performing standard diagnostic tests, the medical herbalist will take a more holistic approach and look for specific clues to help arrive at a diagnosis. Here the herbalist is testing the patient's reflexes.*

Left *Once a diagnosis is reached, the same herbalist will prepare a remedy or remedies from the herbal armoury. The herbalist here is mixing a remedy from herbal tinctures, although powdered herbs or dried plants for use in tea could also be given.*

As well as a combination of herbs specially selected to help the unique health problems of each individual, the patient may leave the consultation room with a list of dietary suggestions or foods to avoid or eat more of.

They may also be recommended relaxation routines to follow or Bach Flower Remedies (*see page* 105) to help emotional factors affecting physical wellbeing. Or perhaps the patient will be sent away with a small growing plant to bring a little love and beauty into their life.

Whatever the remedy, healing is a two-way process and the patient must take responsibility for his or her own health and actively participate in any cure. Those who expect a 'magic pill' to solve their problems with little of their own effort may be happier with orthodox therapies.

Working together

Existing orthodox medication that the patient is taking also needs to be checked. Herbalists would certainly not recommend that you stop taking vital drugs, but any incompatibility of these drugs with herbal remedies must be considered when prescribing plant medicines. Similarly, many patients turn to herbs because they are anxious to phase out their drugs, for whatever reason, and a safe programme for replacing them with gentler herbal remedies needs to be devised, preferably with the support and co-operation of the patient's doctor. Herbal remedies, for example, can be very helpful for sufferers trying to break an addiction to tranquillizers or sleeping pills, or as alternatives for those suffering the side effects from non-steroidal anti-inflammatory drugs used for arthritis.

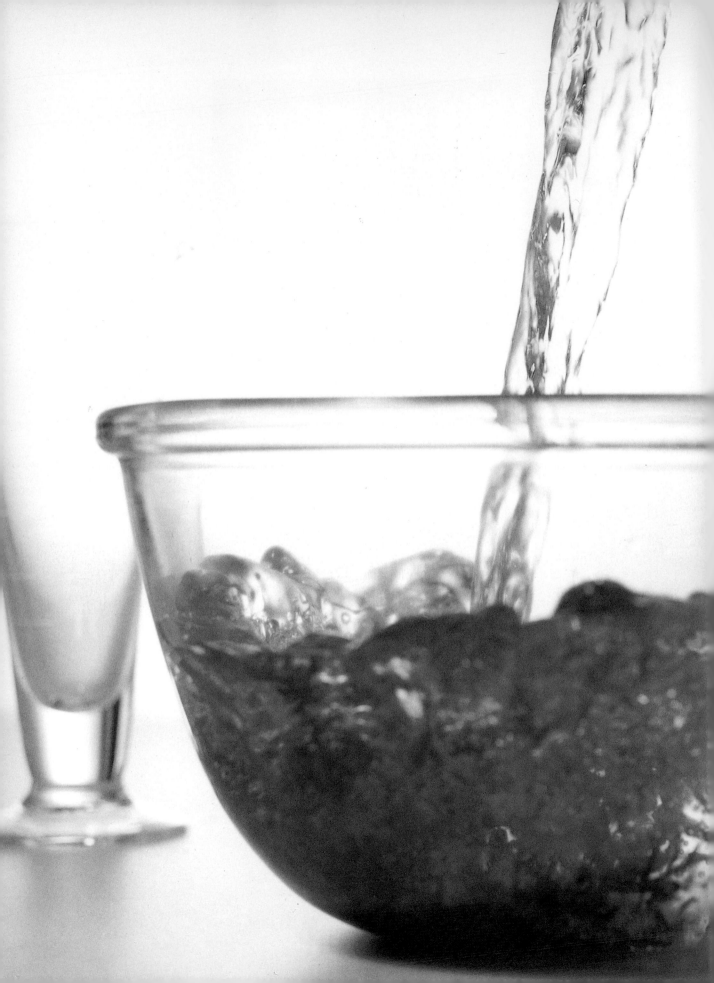

Self-help
with herbs

Making herbal remedies at home, using plants gathered from your own garden or window box, is extremely pleasant and satisfying. It is also very therapeutic: the time spent brewing a relaxing herbal infusion or blending a soothing massage oil is all part of the healing process. This section shows you how to make basic remedies at home, provides details on how to grow your own herbs, and gives you suggestions on what to buy.

Simple remedies, equipment and storage

Chewing fresh herbs may be the simplest way of taking a remedy, but it is rarely palatable or convenient. Before using herbs, you need to extract their active constituents, and traditionally this has been by making teas – soaking the herb in water and then drinking the liquid. Alcohol will also extract these vital chemicals and wine has been used since ancient times to make herbal brews. Today we use tinctures, which are alcohol/water extracts, as these can be more convenient than brewing teas several times a day.

Most herbs are used in combination with up to a dozen different plants included in the mixture. If you are using a single herb then the remedy is often called a 'simple'. When making teas it is generally easier to mix the dried herbs first and then make the remedy; with tinctures it is always best to make a simple tincture and then combine these to make the chosen remedy.

With creams and infused oils, professional herbalists will generally make separate mixtures for each individual herb and then blend them to suit individual needs. For home use though, where a remedy is being made for a specific patient or application, it is often just as easy to mix the dried herbs and make a combined extract.

Using herbs correctly

While herbal medicine is generally regarded as quite safe, many of the plants involved are potentially toxic in high doses and therefore need to be used with caution. Never exceed the stated dose and stop treatment if unexpected symptoms occur or existing ones worsen. Always be certain you are using the correct plant. This is especially important when you are collecting herbs in the wild: comfrey leaves are easily mistaken for foxglove, for example. Use a good wild plant handbook to identify specimens, and if in doubt, don't use it.

Basic equipment

Never use aluminium saucepans or kettles for brewing your herbs as microscopic amounts of the metal may dissolve into the mixture. Always use stainless steel, ceramic or enamelled cookware. Nylon sieves are also more suitable than metal ones and are easier to clean. Use wooden or stainless steel spatulas.

Although you can make most herbal remedies using basic kitchen equipment, a few items are especially useful:

- Double saucepan (double boiler): Ointments and creams need to be heated in a saucepan over water, so a double saucepan is ideal, although you can use a basin on top of a saucepan of water instead.

- Jelly bag: Used in jam making, jelly bags are useful for pressing herbal tinctures, creams, ointments and infused oils if you do not have a wine press.

- Wine press: The type sold for home wine-making is ideal to press out herbal tinctures, creams, ointments, and infused oils.

- A selection of small glass jars and bottles with screw tops for storing creams, oils and tinctures. Use dark glass and choose 30-60 ml/1–2 fl oz ointment pots and 100–200 ml/3½–7 fl oz bottles for infused oils and tinctures. Pots and bottles used for storing mixtures should be completely sterile and airtight.

- Dropping pipette (dropper).

All equipment needs to be kept clean and sterile as herbal mixtures can easily go mouldy during long-term storage if they become contaminated. If making herbal remedies regularly keep a separate set of utensils to avoid contamination with bacteria from food. Otherwise wash the equipment thoroughly in very hot water before using them and dry metal pans and metal spatulas in a hot oven.

Weighing dried herbs

Kitchen scales are generally suitable for weighing out herbs. If using the traditional balance style, ensure that the weights set includes 5 and 10 g weights. Top weighing scales are available with increments of 1, 2, 5, and 10 g; the smaller the increment the greater the degree of accuracy in weighing. Electronic scales are the simplest to use and will generally display weights accurately to 0.1 g. If it is difficult to weigh less than 10 g on your set of scales, then double the quantities given in the remedies section for individual dried herbs in a particular ailment recipe, and divide the resulting mixture in half, reserving a portion for the next day's use.

Measuring liquids

Conical or straight-sided measuring cylinders are best for measuring out tinctures, lotions, and oils. As an alternative you can use a standard measuring jug marked in increments of 5 ml/1 tsp or 10 ml/2 tsp, doubling the quantities given in an individual recipe if necessary to make measuring easier and more accurate. As a guide, 20 drops of liquid falling naturally from a dropping pipette will equal approximately 1 ml, so drops can be used as an alternative if small quantities are required (for example, 50 drops = 2.5 ml).

Sterilizing equipment

Herbal medicines usually keep well, but moulds will develop if non-sterile storage jars and bottles are used. There is rarely a problem with tinctures – the high alcohol content kills many bacteria, but creams and syrups rapidly deteriorate. Sterilization preparations sold for home wine-making or for baby's bottles – usually based on sodium metabisuphite or sodium hypochlorite – are ideal. Soak bottles, jars, and tops in these diluted mixtures for at least 30 minutes (or as directed on the packet), then rinse them with freshly boiled water before drying in a hot oven. Or, wash glass containers thoroughly in freshly boiled water, then put them into a hot oven, at least 160°C/325°F/gas mark 3, for an hour. Handle with care when removing the containers and use when cool. This method is obviously not suitable for plastic containers.

Below Few pieces of special equipment are needed to make and store herbal remedies, other than a selection of bottles and jars and a measuring jug.

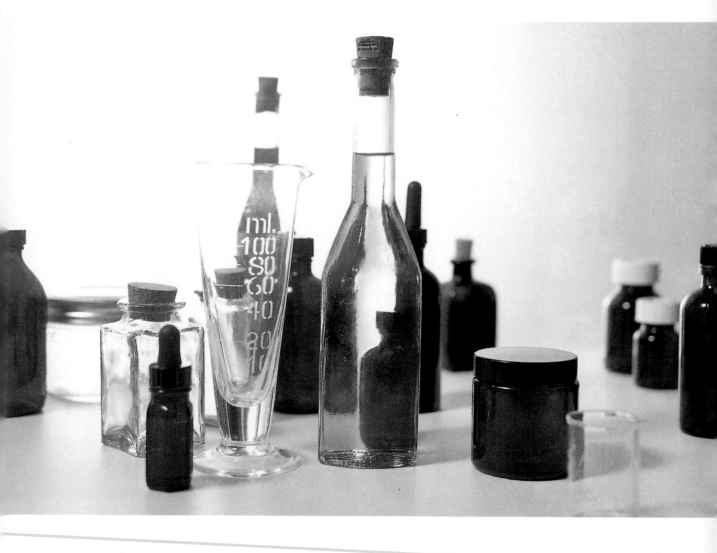

Infusions and decoctions

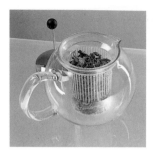
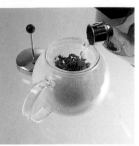
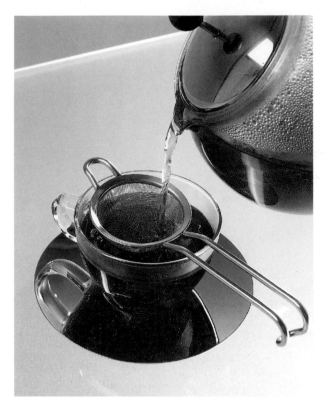

Herbal infusions

Herbal infusions – sometimes called tisanes – are made as you would make tea, except that the usual standard therapeutic dose is 25 g/1 oz of dried herb to ½ litre/1 pint of water that is just off the boil rather than boiling vigorously. Infuse for ten minutes, then strain and drink the infusion in three equal wine glass or cup doses during the day. Infusions are used for the flowers and the leafy parts of plants. If using fresh herbs then triple the quantity (for example, 75 g/3 oz instead of 25 g/1 oz) to take account of the extra water content in the herb. If making individual cups, then you will generally need 1–2 tsp of dried herb per cup.

The infusion should be stored in a covered jug or teapot in a cool place and used within 24 hours.

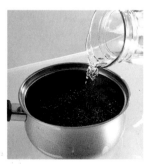
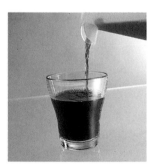

Decoctions

Decoctions are usually made with 25 g/1 oz of herbs to ¾ litre/1½ pints of cold water, brought to the boil and then simmered until the volume has been reduced by about one-third. Drink three wine glass or cup doses during the day. For individual doses, use 1–2 tsp of herb per 1½ cups of water. Decoctions are used in the West for roots, barks, some berries, and the twiggy parts of plants.

In China decoctions, often called 'soups', are always used

instead of infusions with as much as 100 g/4 oz or more of dried herbs heated in ½–1 litre/1–1¾ pints of water. The decoction can be reduced to 250-500 ml (¼–½ litre)/½–1 pint by simmering, and then this concentrated mix can be given in drop dosages, either neat or diluted in water or fruit juice. Strong decoctions can be extremely bitter and unpleasant to taste and this can be a good way of persuading reluctant patients to drink them.

Strong decoctions can be stored in a refrigerator for up to 48 hours, although, if possible, they should be freshly prepared each day.

Combining infusions and decoctions

Many herbal prescriptions use a mixture of the leafy parts of plants and the roots, so it is necessary to use a combination of infusion and decoction techniques to extract the healing components. You can make two separate brews and then combine them. Alternatively, decoct the roots or barks in ¾ litre/1½ pints of water and then pour this decoction on to the dried herbs and infuse for a further ten minutes before straining the entire mix as before.

Washes, juices, macerations and inhalants

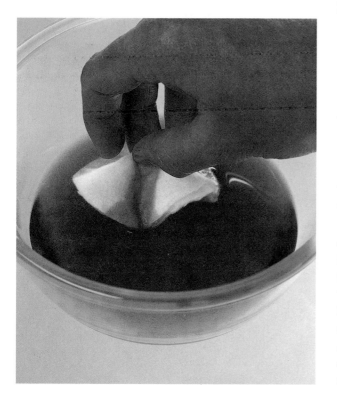

Maceration

Some herbs, such as valerian or marshmallow roots, are best macerated (soaked) in cold water rather than made into an infusion or decoction. Use the same proportions as for an infusion and simply leave the mixture in a cool place overnight. In the morning strain the mix and use as an infusion.

Juices

To prepare herb juices, pulp the plant in a domestic juicer or food processor, and then squeeze the mixture through a jelly bag to obtain the juice. Large quantities of herbs are needed (a 9 litre/ 2 gallon bucket full of fresh herbs may yield only 100 ml/3½ fl oz or less of juice). Juices need to be stored in a refrigerator and should be used within a week. Discard if there are any signs of fermentation.

Steam inhalants

These are ideal for asthma, catarrh and sinusitis (*see pages* 95, 96, 97). Place the herb (usually 1 tbsp of dried herb is sufficient) in a mixing bowl and pour over about 1–2 litres/1¾-3½ pints of boiling water. Cover your head with a towel, bend over the bowl, and inhale for as long as you can bear the heat, or until the mixture cools. Avoid going into a cold atmosphere for at least 30 minutes after the inhalation.

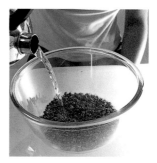

Washes

Infusions or decoctions can be used to bathe wounds, sores, skin rashes, and ulcers. Use cotton wool to apply the wash, bathing from the centre of the wound or sore outwards. A plastic atomizer can be useful to spray rashes or varicose ulcers with the

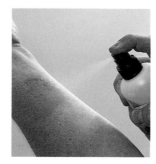

mixture. Sterile and well-strained infusions and decoctions can also be used in eyebaths (*see page* 136).

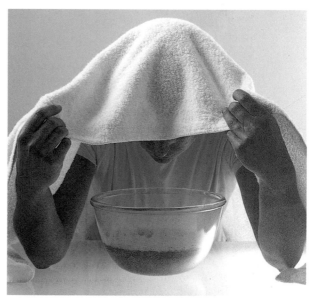

Syrups, wines and tinctures

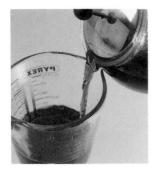

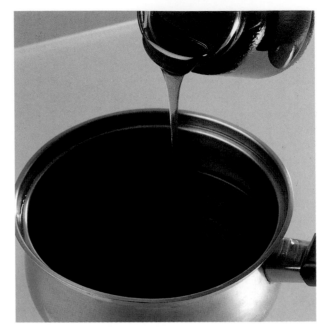

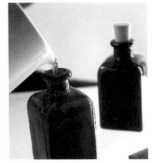

Syrups

Sugar or honey can be used to preserve herbal infusions and decoctions; they are also ideal for cough remedies as the sweetness is soothing.

Make a standard infusion or decoction (depending on herb to be used) as described on page 30. After straining the mixture, make a syrup by adding ½ litre/1½ pints of liquid to 500 g/1 lb of unrefined sugar or honey. Stir the mixture in a cast iron or stainless steel saucepan over heat until the sugar or honey is completely dissolved and the mixture forms a syrup. Allow to cool and then store in clean glass bottles with a cork.

Don't use screw-tops – syrups often ferment and screw-tops can easily cause bottles to explode.

Tonic wines

This is a delightful way to take your medicine and is especially suitable for roots such as *He Shou Wu*, *Dang Gui*, or ginseng. Ideally, you need an old-fashioned vinegar vat (available from kitchen shops), but a large jug (with a lid) or a rum pot can be used instead.

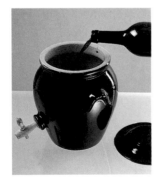

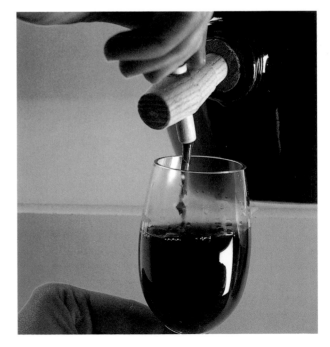

Put 500 g/1 lb of herb into the vat and add 2 litres/3½ pints of good quality wine (preferably red) so that the herb is completely covered, otherwise it will go mouldy. Cover the vat and leave for at least two weeks. Vinegar vats have a tap at the bottom, making it easy to pour off a sherry glass of the liquid for a daily dose.

Top up the mixture with more red wine to keep the herb covered. Replace the herb after two months.

Tinctures

A tincture is an alcoholic extract of the active ingredients in a herb. It is made by soaking the dried or fresh plant material in a mixture of alcohol and water for two weeks and then straining the mix through a wine press or jelly bag.

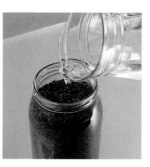

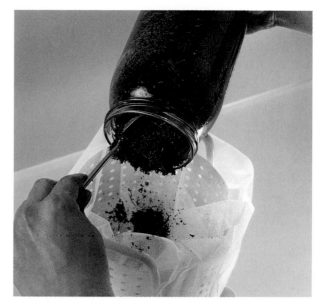

Commercially produced tinctures are usually made from ethyl alcohol. In some countries this is readily available duty free, but in others, such as the United Kingdom, the supply is strictly controlled by H M Customs and Excise, so it is not always easy to obtain low-cost suppliers of ethyl alcohol for home use. Although any alcohol can be used to make tinctures, not all alcohols are safe to drink, so great care needs to be taken with home production. Methyl alcohol is extremely poisonous, and although some suggest using isopropyl alcohol (rubbing alcohol) for tincture-making this, too, can be very toxic. Glycerol, which has the benefit of being very low cost and available from pharmacists, can be used but the resulting tinctures are slightly slimy to the palate. Glycerol tinctures may be preferable for children, pregnant women and also for reformed alcoholics.

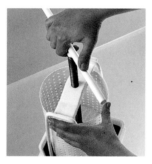

The simplest source of alcohol for home tincture-making is to use ready-made wines and spirits – vodka is ideal as it is contains fewer other flavourings.

Standard herbal tinctures usually contain 25 per cent alcohol in water (25 ml/1 fl oz) of pure alcohol with 75 ml/3 fl oz of water). This is a little weaker than most commercial spirits (usually 37.5 per cent alcohol) so the vodka will need diluting slightly with water (³⁄₄ litres/1¹⁄₂ pints of vodka to 375 ml/15 fl oz of water) to make the required strength. Tinctures made from resinous plants, such as rosemary, are generally 45 per cent alcohol; as it is difficult to obtain this strength for home use, these tinctures may be best bought commercially.

Standard tinctures are usually made in the weight:volume proportion 1:5 (1 kg/2 lb of herb to 5 litres/10 pints of alcohol/water mixture or 500 g/1 lb of herb to 2¹⁄₂ litres/5 pints of liquid). For domestic use using 200 g/8 oz of herb with 1 litre/ 2¹⁄₂ pints of liquid is usually a sufficient quantity to make at one time. If using a fresh herb then you need to triple this quantity

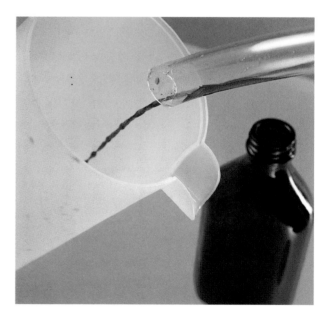

for the water content of the herb (600 g/1¹⁄₂ lb of fresh herb to 1 litre/2¹⁄₂ pints of liquid).

Put the herb into a large jar – such as an old-fashioned glass sweet jar, available from old sweet shops and kitchen shops, or use a catering size mayonnaise jar – and pour over with the alcohol/water mixture. Store in a cool place for two weeks, shaking the mixture each day, then filter it through a wine press or use a jelly bag. Store the tincture in clean, dark glass containers. The herbal residue is an ideal addition to the compost heap.

Tinctures will general last for two years or more without deterioration, although Ayurvedic medicine proposes that the tinctures increase in potency as they age.

Creams and ointments and infused oils

Creams and ointments

Creams are a mixture of oils or fats and water which will be absorbed by the skin, while ointments contain only oils or fats and so form a separate layer over the skin.

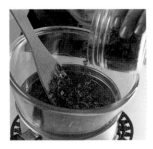

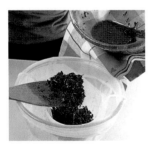

Ointments

Ointments are suitable where the skin is already weak or soft or where some protection is needed from additional moisture, as in nappy rash (*see page* 149). Traditionally ointments were made using animal fats and the simplest method is to heat dried herbs in melted lard or Vaseline for a couple of hours, then strain the mix through a jelly bag or wine press and pour into small jars to set.

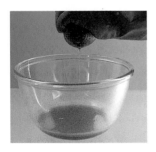

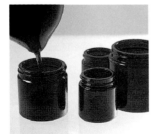

Creams

Creams can easily be made with an emulsifying ointment (available from most large pharmacists), which is a mixture of paraffin oils. This is blended with a proportion of water, glycerol and herbs to make a cream. Heating the dried herb in the mixture will extract its healing chemicals.

To make the cream use 300 g/10 oz of emulsifying ointment, 135 ml/4½ fl oz of glycerol, 165 ml/5½ fl oz of water and 60 g/2¼ oz of dried herb.

Melt the emulsifying ointment over boiling water using a bowl or a double saucepan and then add the rest of the ingredients. Heat for about three hours, topping up the water in the lower pan to prevent it from boiling dry. Strain the mixture through a wine press, jelly bag or fine nylon sieve before it starts to cool, and then stir the cream constantly until it sets. Store in small clean, airtight plastic or glass jars.

You can substitute 300 ml/ 10 fl oz of ready-made herbal tincture (*see page* 35) for the water, glycerol and dried herb mix, and melt the ointment, add the tincture, and continue heating and stirring for a few minutes to combine the two. Remove from the heat and stir the mix until it cools.

Creams made in this way will usually keep for several months, although their shelf-life can be prolonged by storing in a refrigerator or cool larder. This method is suitable for making creams of marigold, comfrey, chickweed, cleavers, lemon balm, chamomile, sage, and melilot.

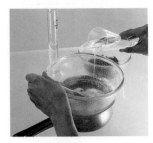

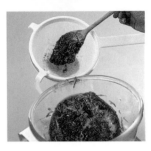

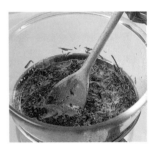

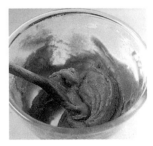

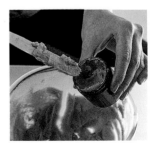

Infused oils

Infused oils can be used for ointments or as massage oils and are an excellent and simple way of using herbs.

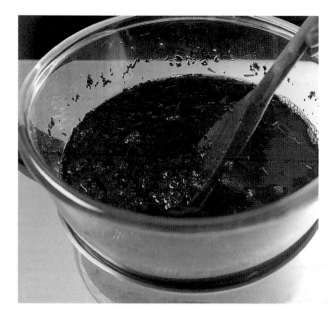

Hot infusion

Heat 100 g/4 oz of dried (300 g/12 oz of fresh) herb in ½ litre/1 pint of sunflower oil (or a similar oil) in a double saucepan for about three hours. Press out the oil through a muslin bag or wine press.

This method is suitable for making infused comfrey, chickweed, nettle, and rosemary oils.

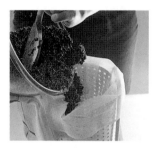

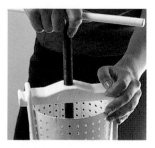

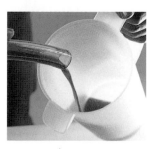

Cold infusion

As the oil is not heated in this method, it is better to use a good quality seed oil that is rich in essential fatty acids, such as gamma-linolenic (GLA) or cis-linoleic acids, which have significant therapeutic properties.

Fill a large jar with the dried herb and completely cover with the oil. Leave the jar on a sunny windowsill or in the greenhouse for at least three weeks. During this time it will gradually change colour – for example, St John's wort oil is a rich red, marigold is orange. Strain the oil through a wine press or jelly bag and then, if possible, repeat the whole process using the fresh herb and the once-infused oil, leaving the mix in a sunny place for a further two or three weeks – this makes a stronger oil. Finally, strain and store in clean, airtight bottles.

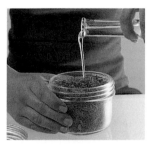

Infused oils will generally last for at least a year, often longer. This method is best for oils made from flowers or flowering tops as in the above examples.

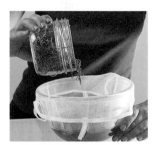

These infused oils can be thickened with beeswax and lanolin to make ointments and creams. For ointments, use 100 ml/4 fl oz of infused oil, 25 g/1 oz beeswax and 25 g/1 oz of anhydrous lanolin (available from pharmacists). Melt the fats and warm the infused oil in a separate double boiler. Mix the two together and stir well. Pour into clean glass jars while still warm and allow to set.

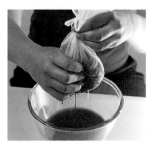

To make a cream, use 100 ml/4 fl oz of infused oil, 25 g/1 oz of beeswax, 25 g/1 oz of anhydrous lanolin and 50 ml/2 fl oz of herbal tincture (*see page* 35). Melt the fats and oil in a double boiler and warm the tincture slightly. Combine the mixtures, stir well, and continue stirring until the mix cools and thickens. Store in clean glass jars.

Combination creams are easy to make using this method – try comfrey and rosemary for arthritic pain (*see page* 131), chamomile and St John's wort for inflammations and melilot and marigold for varicose eczema (*see page* 143).

Massage oils, compresses and poultices

Massage oils

Most essential oils can irritate the skin and are best diluted in a vegetable oil base. Almond or wheatgerm oils are often used, but sunflower oil or even basic vegetable oil used for cooking are also acceptable. Infused oils can be used on their own or as a base to which the essences are added.

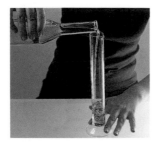

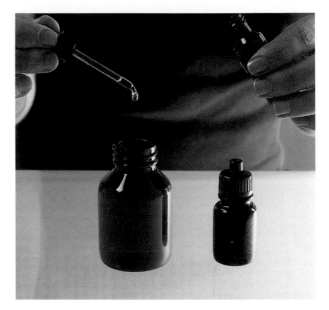

Generally a 5–10 per cent solution of the essential oil in the base is adequate. This means that you use 5–10 ml/1–2 tsp of the essential oil with 90–95 ml/

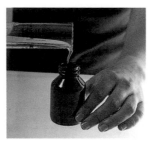

3–3¼ fl oz to make100 ml/4 fl oz of the mixture. As a guide, 1 ml is about 20 drops, so for 10 ml/2 tsp of carrier oil you would need 10–20 drops of essential oil.

A little of the massage oil mixture should be applied directly to the skin and massaged in gently but thoroughly. For

more localized problems, such as the muscles and joints in rheumatism (*see page* 131), you should concentrate the massage on the affected area. Chest rubs should obviously be focused on the thorax, while relaxing or tonic mixtures can be used in whole body massage.

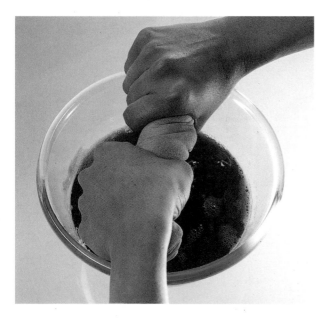

Compresses

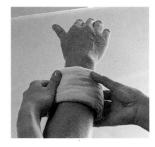

Compresses help to speed up the healing process, as with wounds or muscle injuries. They are basically cloth pads soaked in herbal extracts and usually applied when hot to painful limbs, swellings, and strains. Use a clean piece of cotton, cotton wool, linen or surgical gauze soaked in a hot, strained infusion, decoction or tincture (dilute 10 ml/2 tsp with 100 ml/4 fl oz of hot water) and apply to the affected area. When the compress cools repeat the process using a fresh, hot mixture. Hot compresses can also be used to help draw pus from boils or abscesses (*see page* 128). Occasionally a cold compress may be used, for example, with some types of headaches when a cool pad soaked in lavender infusion may be suitable.

Poultices

Poultices have a very similar action to compresses, but they involve applying the whole herb directly to an affected area rather than using a liquid extract. Poulticing was a favourite household remedy in days

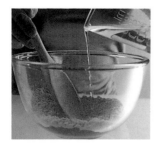

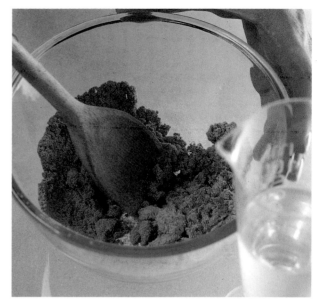

gone by, with bread or mashed potato used as the carrying mixture for a herbal infusion or oil. Like compresses, hot poultices can be used for swellings, sprains, or to draw pus or splinters (*see pages* 128 *and* 147), but cold pastes/poultices can also be useful, as with comfrey root applied to varicose ulcers. A much simpler method of poulticing than soaking bread or potato in a herbal infusion is to sweat the herb in a saucepan with very little water, then strain it and spread the mixture onto gauze and apply this

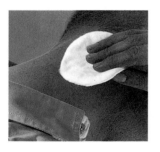

to the affected area. Hold the poultice in place with a plaster or loose bandage.

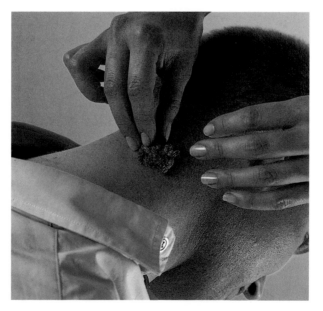

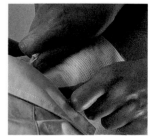

Powdered herbs can also be used to make poultices: all you have to do is mix the powder with a little hot water to form a paste and then spread directly on to the affected area or on to gauze as before.

If you are applying poultices directly to the skin, you should grease the skin first with a little vegetable oil to prevent it from sticking.

When you use a hot poultice, make sure to renew it each time it cools.

Growing and buying herbs

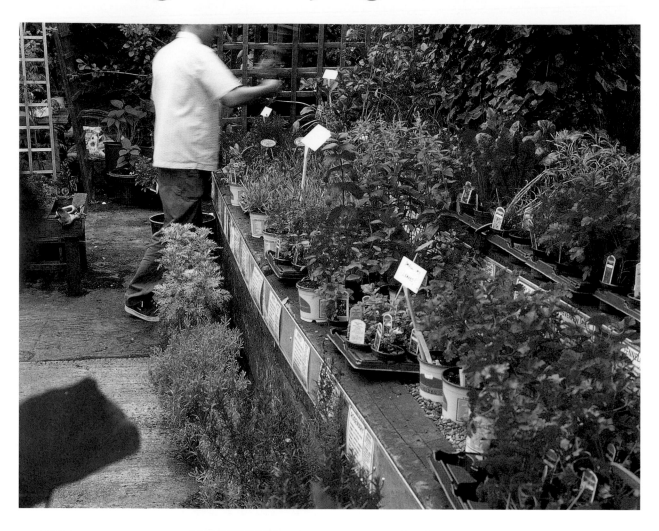

Growing herbs

There is really nothing nicer than being able to go to your own garden or window box and snip a few herbs for a therapeutic tea or to turn into a healing ointment. Home grown and freshly dried herbs also tend to be far more potent than commercial specimens which may have been stored for many months before sale. Growing herbs is no more difficult than cultivating any other sort of herbaceous plants or shrubs and they will also provide a constant array of healing aromas to enjoy in your garden.

For the less common medicinal herbs, home cultivation can also be the most practical way to ensure a continual supply of needed plants. Obviously, use of chemical pesticides should be avoided for any herbs intended for medicinal use.

It is generally easiest to buy perennial herb plants from a specialist nursery or to take cuttings, but biennial and annual

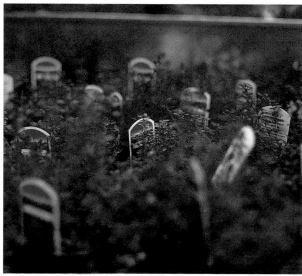

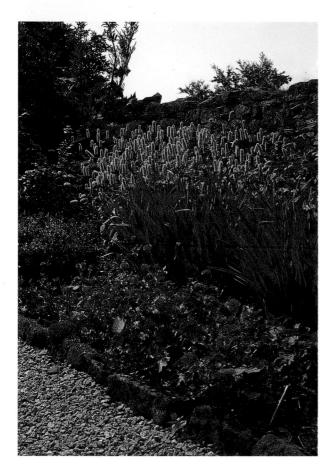

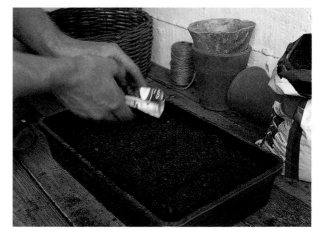

Opposite above *Specialist nurseries stock an enormous range of herbs to grow and then use in your remedies. Perennial plants are best bought, but you can grow biennials and annuals from seed.*

Opposite below *Thyme makes a superb digestive remedy, as well as being an antiseptic and expectorant.*

Above *This lush herb garden features bistort among other herbs.*

Above right *Lavender can be grown not only for its medicinal properties but also for its lovely scent.*

Right *Perennial and most biennial herb seeds can be raised in seed trays.*

ones are best grown from seed. Annual medicinal and salad herbs to sow regularly include basil, borage, Californian poppy, German chamomile, dill and pot marigold. Although a biennial, parsley should be sown annually, ideally in the place where it is intended to grow as it does not transplant well. Pour freshly boiled water over the newly planted parsley seeds to encourage rapid germination. Other biennials readily grown from seed include mullein and melilot.

Many herbs will self-seed enthusiastically, which can be both a very useful source of new plants and also a real nuisance, demanding ruthless weeding out. Particular culprits here include fennel, lady's mantle, feverfew, lemon balm, melilot, mullein and skullcap.

Some herbs are normally in the 'garden weeds' category, so don't consign them all to the compost heap. Useful weeds include dandelion, red clover, shepherd's purse and ground ivy.

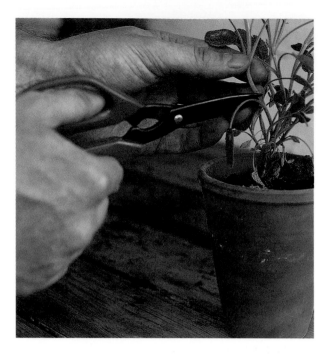

signs of the zodiac. The main considerations for modern herb gatherers, however, are to collect the herbs on a dry day, and to ensure the plant is at the peak of maturity when the concentration of active ingredients is highest.

- Flowers: These should be collected when fully open and handled carefully as they are easily damaged. Small flowers (like lavender) can be dried on their stems, but if the stem is fleshy – like mullein – the flowers must be removed and dried individually.

- Leaves: Large leaves (such as burdock) can be gathered individually, but smaller ones (like lemon balm) are best collected on the stem. Leaves of deciduous herbs should generally be gathered just before flowering; evergreen ones like rosemary can be gathered throughout the year. Sometimes young leaves are collected separately for cooking or spring tonics (for example nettles or dandelions for soups and salads). A second crop of the herb can then be taken closer to flowering for the more mature leaves.

Harvesting herbs

The time when herbs are gathered can significantly affect the constituent chemicals and thus their therapeutic properties. In the past complex rituals were followed so that herbs were gathered at the height of their potency – at a certain phase of the moon, when the dog star could be seen, or during particular

- Aerial parts: If using all the aerial parts then the best time to collect is in the midst of flowering, giving a mixture of leaves, stem, flowers and seed head. Skullcap, for example, can be collected when around half of the flowers have formed the characteristic cap-shaped pod.

Above To take cuttings, snip a suitable stem, or break off a piece to give a heel, dip into hormone rooting powder and plant in a small pot in good quality compost.

Right When buying plants from a nursery, look for healthy root growth and avoid plants which are obviously pot-bound or have loose compost. Inspect young plants for signs of disease and avoid any with yellowing leaves.

Opposite Keep fresh dried herbs out of direct sunlight to preserve their potency, aroma, and colour.

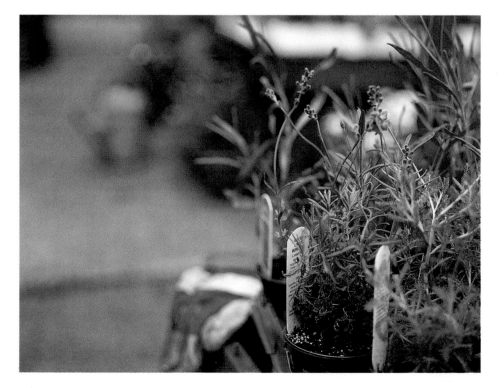

- Seeds: These should be collected when ripe, or with large seed heads like fennel, when around two-thirds of the seeds on a particular head are ripe and before too many have been dispersed by birds or the wind.

- Fruit: Berries and other fruits should be gathered when just ripe and before the fruit becomes too soft or pulpy to dry effectively.

- Root: Roots are generally gathered in the autumn when the aerial parts of the plant have died down and before the ground becomes too hard, making digging difficult. An exception is dandelion, where the roots should be gathered in the spring.

- Bark: This is generally best collected in the autumn when the sap is falling in order to minimize damage to the plant. Never remove all the bark – or a band of bark completely surrounding a tree – unless you want to sacrifice the plant to herbal medicine.

Drying herbs

Herbs need to be dried as quickly as possible and away from bright sunlight to preserve the aromatic ingredients and prevent oxidation of other chemicals. Good air circulation is also needed, so make only small bunches or leave the airing cupboard door open if you are using that as your drying space. A dry garden shed with a low-powered fan running can be effective, but avoid drying herbs in garages as they can become contaminated with petrol fumes.

In warm conditions with a good air circulation it is possible to dry herbs completely within five or six days, sometimes even less. The longer the plant takes to dry the more likely it is to discolour and lose its flavour. Ideally the temperature in the drying room should be between 20°–32°C/70°–90°F and should never go above 38°C/100.2°F.

Label dried herbs with the variety, source, and date – most should keep for 12–18 months without significant deterioration if they are dried and stored correctly.

Buying herbs

When buying dried herbs, look for those that are stored away from bright sunlight and have a good colour. Herbs rapidly fade, and if they look drab and brown they may well be past their prime.

Always buy from a reputable supplier to ensure good quality and accurate labelling. Plants can be and indeed often are wrongly labelled – in garden centres as well as in herb shops –

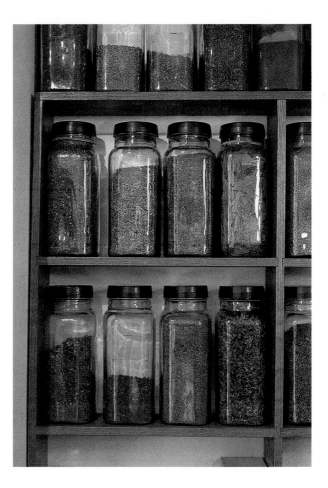

and unless you have a good idea of the correct appearance, smell or taste, then the mistake can lead to the totally wrong remedies being produced.

Today there are also many ready-made, over-the-counter, herbal remedies to choose from. Some of these are licensed and thus can give an indication of their therapeutic use and properties. Others are sold as food supplements or as simple unlicensed herbs and by law, can give no indication on the packaging of recommended use.

If you are in doubt you should ask a pharmacist or health food store assistant, or check in your own herbal before going out to buy.

Storing herbs

Herbs should always be stored in clean, dry, airtight containers, away from direct sunlight. Dried herbs soon deteriorate in bright sunlight, so it is important to use dark glass or pottery containers. Tinctures, infused oils and essential oils should also be kept in dark glass bottles. When you are blending them you should only make enough to last for two or three weeks to avoid wastage and deterioration.

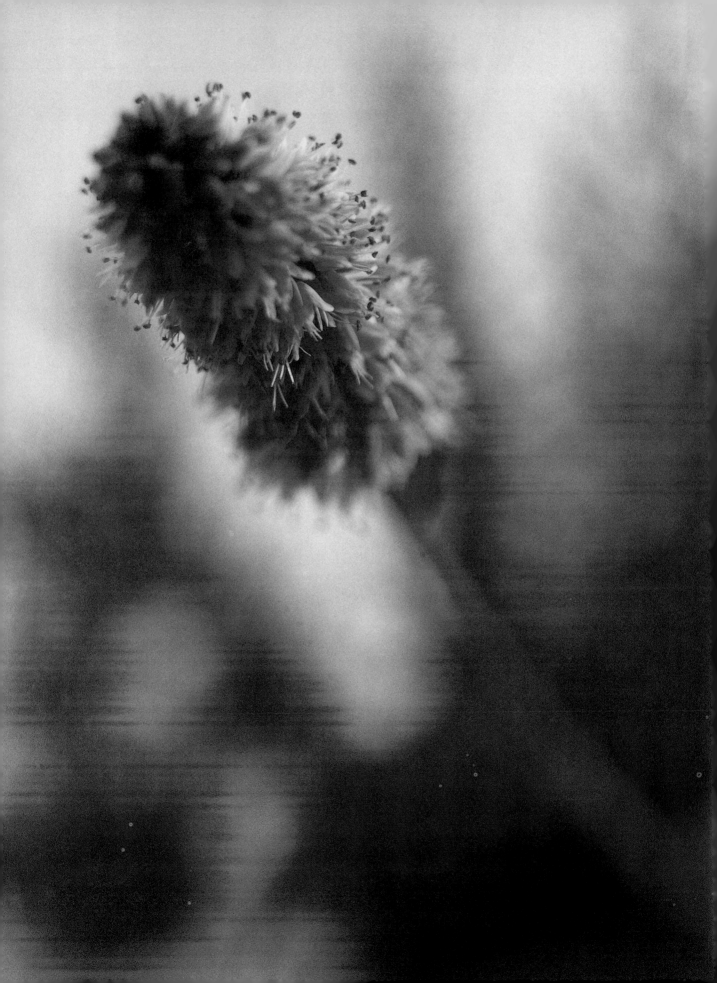

Using herbs for
health

There are many thousands of herbs in regular use worldwide and any selection inevitably has to omit many hundreds of helpful plants. A few herbs – such as blue cohosh or bugleweed – have very specific actions and thus a limited number of uses. Others, like marigold and chamomile, have a broader spectrum of properties and are suitable for very diverse complaints. In this section we detail 120 popular healing herbs which will generally be readily available in shops or for growing at home.

Yarrow *Achillea millefolium*

A common meadow herb, with the country name 'nosebleed', yarrow is used in remedies for colds, hay fever and catarrh. As a diuretic, it can also be used for urinary problems and to counter fluid retention (*see page* 111) or to reduce blood pressure (*see page* 90).

Parts used: Leaves, flowers, essential oil

Actions: *Aerial parts/flowers:* Astringent, diaphoretic, peripheral vasodilator, digestive stimulant, restorative for menstrual system, febrifuge.
Essential oil: Anti-inflammatory, antiallergenic, antispasmodic

Used in: Infusions, tinctures, massage rubs

Cautions: A uterine stimulant, so avoid in pregnancy. The fresh plant can sometimes cause contact dermatitis and, rarely, may increase the skin's photosensitivity

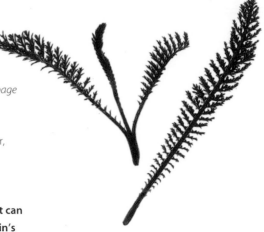

Buchu *Agathosma betulina*

Buchu originated in South Africa where it was traditionally used as an external dusting powder to protect the skin. It has a distinctive blackcurrant flavour and is a popular remedy for cystitis (*see page* 114) and fluid retention (*see page* 114).

Parts used: Leaves

Actions: Diuretic, diaphoretic and stimulant; tonic and warming for the kidneys

Used in: Infusions, tinctures, capsules

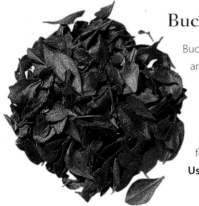

Agrimony *Agrimonia eupatoria*

Agrimony is an astringent, bitter herb useful for diarrhoea (*see page* 121) and to stop bleeding. It has a long tradition as a wound herb and was the main ingredient of 'arquebusade water', a 15th-century remedy for battlefield gunshot wounds. Agrimony is also diuretic and contains silica, which makes it a good healing remedy for urinary disorders.

Parts used: Aerial parts/leaves

Actions: Astringent, diuretic, tissue healer, stops bleeding, bile stimulant, some antiviral activity reported

Used in: Infusions, tinctures

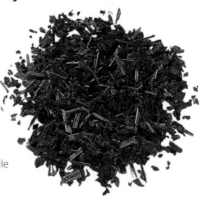

Lady's mantle *Alchemilla xanthoclora* ♡ ❀ ♀

Lady's mantle is rich in tannins, and so it is a good astringent, and it is also useful for diarrhoea, sore throats (*see page* 97), skin sores and weeping dermatitis. It also has a gynaecological action and is used in parts of Europe as a menstrual regulator – especially for heavy periods (*see page* 112) or in ointments for vaginal itching.

Parts used: Aerial parts, leaves

Actions: Astringent, menstrual regulator, digestive tonic, anti-inflammatory, wound herb

Used in: Infusions, tinctures, ointments, gargles, pessaries

Caution: Avoid high doses in pregnancy as it is a uterine stimulant

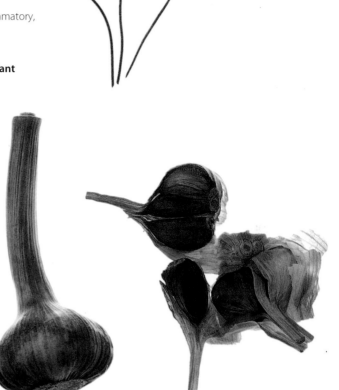

Garlic *Allium sativa* ♡ ❀ ⬭ ⬤ ◖ ⬤

Familiar as a food flavouring, garlic has been used for treating colds (*see page* 126) and catarrh (*see page* 96) since ancient Egyptian times. Modern research has also confirmed its role in treating heart and circulatory problems (*see pages* 89–90).

Parts used: Clove, oil

Actions: Antibiotic, expectorant, diaphoretic, hypotensive, antithrombotic, hypolipidaemic, hypoglycaemic, antihistamine, antiparasitic

Used in: Capsules/tablets, ointments, syrups, raw in cooking

Cautions: Can irritate weak stomachs and sensitive skins. Avoid high doses in pregnancy and during breastfeeding

Aloe *Aloe vera* ♡ ⬤ ◖ ⬤

While 'bitter aloes' is a purgative extract made from various species of aloe, aloe vera yields a mucilaginous (sticky) gel that is largely used externally as a wound healer and to relieve burns and skin inflammations, including eczema and thrush (*see page* 114). The gel is also made into a variety of popular over-the-counter remedies, which are promoted as tonics and restoratives. A tropical plant, it can be grown as a houseplant in temperate climates.

Parts used: Sap, leaves

Actions: Purgative, bile stimulant, wound healer, tonic, demulcent, antifungal, styptic, sedative, anthelmintic

Used in: Ointments, tonic wines, tinctures, capsules

Cautions: Avoid in pregnancy as it is strongly purgative. High doses of leaf extracts may cause vomiting

Galangal *Alpinia officinarum*

Galangal was introduced to Europe by Arab physicians more than 1000 years ago. Traditionally it is used as a warming, digestive remedy and for travel sickness (*see page* 152) and is very similar to ginger. It can also be used to relieve the symptoms of angina pectoris and minor heart disorders.

Parts used: Rhizomes, oil

Actions: Bitter, stimulant, carminative, antiemetic, antifungal, warming

Used in: Tinctures, decoctions, capsules

Marshmallow *Althaea officinale*

Marshmallow can be used for bronchitis (*see page* 95), irritating coughs, and cystitis (*see page* 114). The root is especially soothing for the digestive system, and so it is ideal for gastritis and heartburn (*see pages* 120, 121). Externally it is used for various skin problems and has a soothing, softening effect on the skin.

Parts used: Root, leaves, flowers

Actions: *Root and leaves:* Demulcent, expectorant, diuretic, wound herb

Flowers: Expectorant

Used in: Syrups, infusions, decoctions, tinctures, poultices, ointments

Dill *Anethum graveolens*

Dill is the classic ingredient in baby's gripe water: it is carminative and soothing for the stomach and is an ideal remedy for colic and flatulence (*see page* 149, 123). The seeds can be chewed to relieve bad breath and it can also help reduce menstrual cramps.

Parts used: Seeds, essential oil, leaves

Actions: Carminative, antispasmodic, increases milk production

Used in: Infusions, tinctures, chew raw seeds

Dang Gui (Chinese angelica) *Angelica polymorpha* var. *sinensis*

In China, *Dang Gui* is regarded as the most important tonic herb after ginseng. It is used as a blood tonic for anaemia (*see page* 92), menstrual problems (*see pages* 111–112), or after childbirth (*see page* 117), and is also a mild laxative, especially suitable for the elderly. It is sometimes sold as '*Tang Kwai*' in the West, using an older system of Chinese transliteration.

Part used: Rhizome

Actions: Blood tonic, circulatory stimulant, laxative, antispasmodic, some antibacterial action

Used in: Decoctions, tinctures, tonic wines, capsules

Caution: Avoid in pregnancy

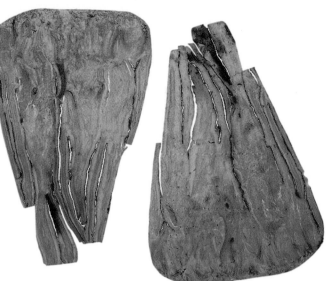

Celery *Apium graveolens*

Celery encourages the excretion of uric acid which is helpful in a number of arthritic conditions, especially gout (*see page* 113). The root was once used for urinary stones (*see page* 109), although now we tend to use mainly the seeds, while a juice made from the stalks has some tonic action for debilitating conditions.

Parts used: Seeds, essential oil

Actions: Antirheumatic, sedative, urinary antiseptic, antispasmodic, diuretic, carminative, hypotensive, some antifungal activity reported

Used in: Juices, infusions, tinctures, powders

Cautions: Celery seed contains bergapten which can increase the photosensitivity of the skin. The oil and high doses of seed should be avoided in pregnancy

Burdock *Arctium lappa*

Burdock root has long been used as a cleansing herb for skin and rheumatic problems (*see page* 131) or where a sluggish digestion is contributing to a build-up of toxins. In China the seeds are traditionally used for treating feverish colds, and modern research does suggest some antimicrobial activity.

Parts used: Leaves, root, seeds

Actions: *Root:* Cleansing, mild laxative, diuretic, diaphoretic, antirheumatic, antiseptic, antibiotic; *Leaves:* Mild laxative, diuretic; *Seeds:* Febrifuge, anti-inflammatory, antibacterial, hypoglycaemic

Used in: Infusions, decoctions, tinctures, poultices

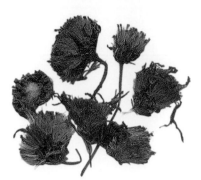

Arnica   *Arnica montana*

Arnica encourages tissue repair after injury so it is ideal after surgery or for sprains (*see page* 133) and bruises. Internally it acts as a circulatory stimulant but is extremely toxic and is generally used only in dilute homeopathic doses.

Parts used: Flowers, rhizome

Actions: Anti-inflammatory, healing, circulatory stimulant

Used in: Ointments, creams, compresses, homeopathic tablets and extracts

Cautions: Only take in homeopathic doses internally. Do not use on open wounds. It may occasionally cause contact dermatitis

Wormwood   *Artemisia absinthum*

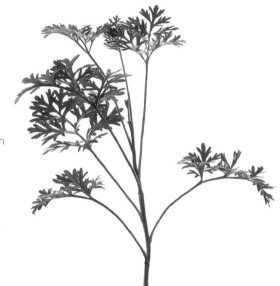

A bitter herb that stimulates digestion, wormwood once formed the key flavouring in the alcoholic drink, *absinthe*, which was popular in the 19th century, although it has now been banned because of its toxicity. Fresh pressed juices and infusions are, however, quite safe to use. Wormwood can help to stimulate gastric function and to improve appetite.

Parts used: Aerial parts

Actions: Bitter digestive tonic, uterine stimulants, anthelmintics

Used in: Infusions, juices

Cautions: Wormwood contains thujone which is a toxic and addictive hallucinogen, so it should only be used for short periods. Avoid in pregnancy and if epileptic

Huang Qi (Milk vetch)

Astragalus membranaceous

An important Chinese tonic herb used to strengthen the body's defences, *Huang Qi* is now being used in the West as an immune stimulant in AIDS treatment and for recurrent infections. The Chinese prefer astragalus root to ginseng as a tonic for the under-40s.

Part used: Root

Actions: Immune stimulant, diuretic, tonic, vasodilator, antipyretic, antiviral

Used in: Decoctions, tinctures, capsules/tablets, chew fried root

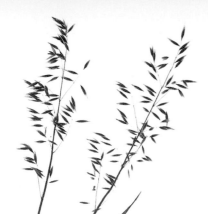

Wild oats *Avena sativa*

Oats have been used as a staple food in northern Europe for centuries. The plant is also a good nerve tonic and restorative, and more recently it has been shown to reduce blood cholesterol levels. Oatmeal is often used externally in skin remedies, while oat straw was a medieval remedy for rheumatism (*see page* 131).

Parts used: Seeds, straw, bran, whole unripe plant

Actions: Antidepressant, restorative nerve tonic, diaphoretic, nutritive; Oatbran is antithrombotic, and reduces cholesterol levels

Used in: Tinctures, porridge, poultices, juice, tablets

Borage *Borago officinalis*

Borage stimulates the adrenal glands to produce adrenaline – the 'flight or fight' hormone which we make in moments of stress. It is also mildly sedative and an antidepressant. The juice can be used externally to soothe itching skin, while the seeds are now known to contain gamma-linolenic acid (GLA) – an essential fatty acid needed for various bodily functions. Borage oil is sometimes marketed as starflower oil.

Parts used: Seed oil, leaves, flowers, juice

Actions: *Leaves:* Adrenal stimulant, stimulates milk flow, diuretic, febrifuge, antirheumatic, diaphoretic, expectorant; *Juice:* Antidepressant, topical antipruritic, demulcent, and anti-inflammatory; *Seeds:* Important source of essential fatty acids

Used in: Infusions, tinctures, capsules, juices

Caution: Use is restricted in some countries

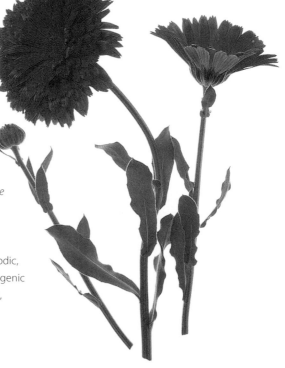

Marigold (Pot marigold) *Calendula officinalis*

Marigold is familiar in patent calendula creams used for dry skin and eczema (*see page* 143), but it is also a powerful menstrual regulator,and digestive remedy. As an antifungal it is helpful for vaginal thrush (*see page* 114) and athlete's foot (*see page* 145); it is also detoxifying and helpful in chronic infections.

Parts used: Flowers, essential oil

Actions: Astringent, antiseptic, antifungal, anti-inflammatory, antispasmodic, wound herb, menstrual regulator, immune stimulant, diaphoretic, oestrogenic

Used in: Infusions, tinctures, infused oils, creams, ointments, compresses, mouthwashes, pessaries

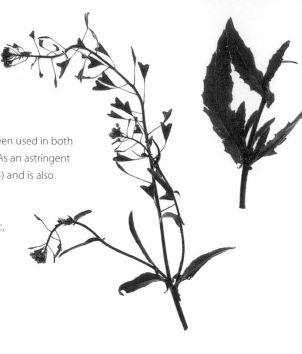

Shepherd's purse *Capsella bursa-pastoris*

Shepherd's purse is a persistent garden weed, but has long been used in both Western and Chinese herbal traditions to stop haemorrhage. As an astringent and urinary antiseptic it is ideal for severe cystitis (*see page* 114) and is also used to normalize heavy menstrual flow (*see page* 112).

Parts used: Leaves, aerial parts

Actions: Astringent, uterine relaxant, styptic, urinary antiseptic, circulatory stimulant, hypotensive

Used in: Infusions, tinctures, poultices, compresses

Caution: Avoid high doses in pregnancy, except during labour, as it stimulates uterine contractions

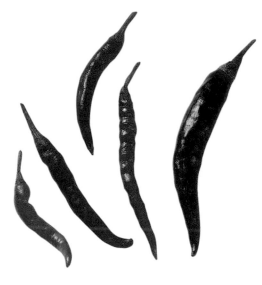

Cayenne *Capsicum frutescens*

The spicy flavouring in West Indian and Eastern cooking, chili or cayenne has been used in Europe since the 16th century as a warming stimulant to improve the circulation (*see* Chilblains *and* Poor circulation, *pages* 93, 91) and also to combat chills.

Part used: Fruit

Actions: Circulatory stimulant, tonic, antispasmodic, diaphoretic, gastric stimulant, carminative, antiseptic, antibacterial, analgesic. Used topically as a counter-irritant and rubefacient

Used in: Infused oils, ointments, tinctures, gargles, massage oils, compresses, infusions, powders, capsules/tablets

Cautions: Avoid in stomach ulceration, pregnancy, and breastfeeding. Do not eat seeds on their own and avoid touching eyes or cuts after handling fresh chili

Blue cohosh *Caulophyllum thalictroides*

Known as 'squaw root' in North America because of its traditional role in treating various gynaecological problems, blue cohosh is still largely used as a menstrual regulator and to ease uterine and ovarian pain (*see* Fibroids, *page* 113).

Parts used: Root and rhizome

Actions: Anti-inflammatory, antispasmodic, uterine stimulant, diuretic, menstrual stimulant, antirheumatic, diaphoretic, uterine tonic

Used in: Decoctions, tinctures

Caution: Avoid in pregnancy, except during labour, as it is a uterine stimulant

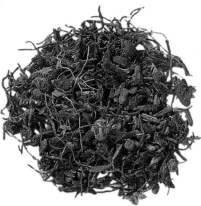

Cornflower *Centaurea cyanus*

Cornflower contains a bitter compound (centaurine)
which accounts for its use as a digestive stimulant (*see*
Indigestion, acidity, *and* heartburn, *page* 121), and the herb is
still included in teas for indigestion in many parts of Europe. An
infusion of the flowers is also a traditional folk remedy for tired eyes –
use a cool, dilute well-strained infusion in an eyebath (*see page* 136).
The seeds have been used for childhood constipation.
Parts used: Flowers, seeds
Actions: Astringent, anti-inflammatory, bitter, mild diuretic
Used in: Infusions, tinctures, eyebaths

Gotu kola *Centella asiatica*

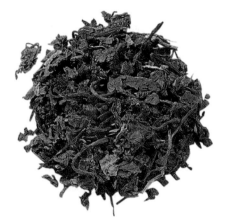

Known in India as *brahmi*, gotu kola is one of the most
important Ayurvedic tonic herbs, long used as a rejuvenating
remedy, and to counter the problems of old age and improve
failing memory.
Parts used: Aerial parts
Actions: Tonic, antirheumatic, peripheral vasodilator, diuretic,
sedative, bitter, laxative
Used in: Infusions, tinctures, powders, poultices

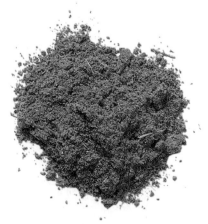

Helonias *Chamaelirium luteum*

Another of the traditional Native American herbs, helonias was used by tribes in
Arkansas for treating ulcers, diarrhoea, and urinary problems. It is mainly used in
the West for gynaecological disorders, including ovarian cysts and menopausal
problems (*see page* 115). This herb is also known as false unicorn root.
Part used: Root
Actions: Uterine and ovarian tonic, menstrual stimulant, diuretic,
oestrogenic, bitter
Used in: Tinctures, decoctions, capsules

Fringe tree · *Chionanthus virginianum*

Fringe tree was used for malaria and as a wound herb by Native Americans, but it is now considered as a highly effective liver and gall bladder remedy for jaundice, gallstones (*see page* 123), hepatitis and poor liver function (*see page* 124).

Part used: Root bark

Actions: Liver stimulant, bile stimulant, laxative, diuretic, tonic

Used in: Decoctions, tinctures, capsules

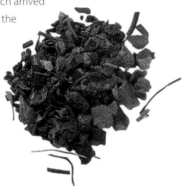

Black cohosh · *Cimicifuga racemosa*

Black cohosh is another of the traditional North American herbs which arrived in Europe in the 19th century. Little is known of its constituents, but the plant has been used to treat ailments as diverse as period pain (*see page* 112) whooping cough, and rheumatism (*see page* 131). It is also popular in menopausal remedies.

Part used: Root

Actions: Sedative, anti-inflammatory, diuretic, antitussive, menstrual stimulant, hypotensive, hypoglycaemic

Used in: Decoctions, tinctures, capsules

Cautions: Excess can cause nausea and vomiting. Avoid in pregnancy

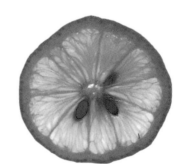

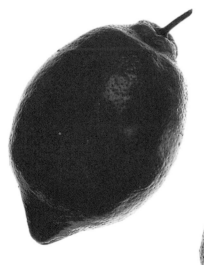

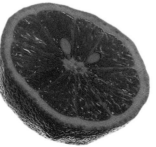

Lemon · *Citrus limon*

Traditionally used in southern Europe to combat major epidemic diseases, lemon is an ideal home remedy to relieve colds, flu and associated symptoms. It is also a good preventative for stomach and circulatory problems.

Parts used: Fruit, essential oil

Actions: Antibacterial, anti-inflammatory, antihistamine, antiviral, antiscorbutic, antioxidant, reduces fever

Used in: Juices, syrups, massage oils

Myrrh *Commiphora myrrha*

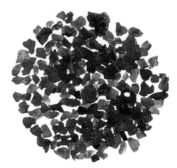

Myrrh resin is extracted from trees in the desert scrublands of northern Somalia, Arabia and the Yemen. It is strongly antiseptic and is often used as a mouthwash or gargle for tonsillitis, mouth ulcers and gum disease.

Part used: Oleo-gum resin

Actions: Antiseptic, stimulant, anti-inflammatory, astringent, expectorant, carminative, antispasmodic

Used in: Tinctures, capsules, gargles and mouthwashes, powders, steam inhalations

Caution: Avoid in pregnancy

Hawthorn

Crataegus laevigata; C. monogyna

Hawthorn is widely used as a cardiac tonic and will improve peripheral circulation (*see* Poor circulation, *page* 91), regulate heart rate and blood pressure and improve coronary blood flow (*see* Atherosclerosis, *page* 89). As an astringent it was more often used in the past for sore throats and diarrhoea.

Parts used: Flowering tops, berries

Actions: Cardiotonic, vasodilator, relaxant, antispasmodic, regulates blood pressure, diuretic

Used in: Infusions, decoction, tinctures, capsules

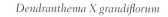

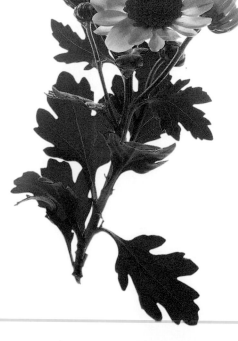

Ju Hua (Chrysanthemum)

Dendranthema X grandiflorum

Popular as a cooling and calming tea in China, these flowers will also reduce high blood pressure. The tea is given for feverish colds and it can help to clear liver stagnation.

Parts used: Flowerheads

Actions: Cooling, febrifuge, diaphoretic, antiseptic, hypotensive

Used in: Infusions, tinctures, powders, poultices

Wild yam   *Dioscorea villosa*

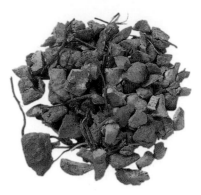

Wild yam, which is rich in steroidal saponins, was the original source of the oral contraceptive pill. It is largely used for colic and rheumatism, but it can also be taken for period pain, cramps, asthma, gastritis and gall bladder problems (*see page* 123).

Parts used: Root and rhizome

Actions: Relaxant for smooth muscles, antispasmodic, bile stimulant, anti-inflammatory, mild diaphoretic

Used in: Decoctions, tinctures

Cautions: May cause nausea in high doses. Avoid high doses in pregnancy

Echinacea (Purple coneflower)

Echinacea spp (E. pallida, E. purpurea. E. angustifolia)

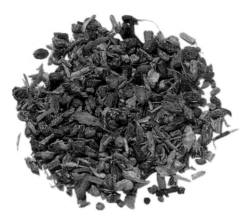

Probably the most important herbal antibiotic in use today, echinacea is a North American plant which has been studied in the West since the 1930s. Although the root has generally been used, recent German research suggests that the aerial parts of *E. purpurea* have similar properties, which is good news for those growing the herb at home. It can combat all types of infections, and is readily available from health food stores.

Parts used: Root, aerial parts

Actions: Antibiotic, immune stimulant, antiallergenic, lymphatic tonic, anti-inflammatory, diaphoretic, wound healer

Used in: Capsules/tablets, tinctures, decoctions, ointments, creams, infusions

Siberian ginseng   *Eleutherococcus senticosus*

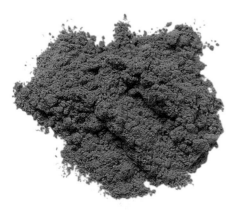

Siberian ginseng came to fame in the 1950s when it was extensively used by Soviet athletes to increase stamina and enhance performance. The herb's main application is as a tonic, helping the body to cope with increased stress levels, and to provide extra energy.

Part used: Root

Actions: Tonic, stimulant, combats stress, antiviral, hypoglycaemic, immune stimulant

Used in: Decoctions, tinctures, capsules

Caution: Do not exceed standard dose or take for prolonged periods

Horsetail *Equisetum arvense* 🌿 ♂ ♀ ♡ 🌿

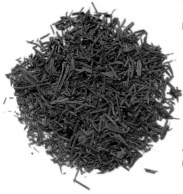

Horsetails grew in prehistoric times and their decayed remains form much of the world's coal seams. The plants are rich in silica, which is very healing, and have largely been used for urinary tract problems (*see* Cystitis, *page* 114), including prostate disorders (*see pages* 108–109). It can also be helpful in deep-seated lung problems, including chronic bronchitis (*see page* 95).

Parts used: Aerial parts, juice

Actions: Astringent, styptic, diuretic, anti-inflammatory, tissue healer

Used in: Decoctions, tinctures, juices, capsules

Californian poppy *Eschscholtzia californica*
🔥 ♡ 🌿

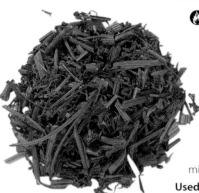

Although a member of the poppy family, Californian poppy – also known as nightcap – is only a mild soporific (*see* Insomnia, *page* 104), suitable even for sleepless children. It can also help to relieve pain.

Parts used: Aerial parts

Actions: Sedative, nerve relaxant, anodyne, mild hypnotic

Used in: Infusions, capsules

Eucalyptus *Eucalyptus globulus*
🌿 🌿 🚫

Originally an Aboriginal remedy, eucalyptus arrived in Europe in the 19th century and has been used as a potent antiseptic for infections ever since. The diluted oil makes a good rub for aching muscles and joints. Fresh leaves from garden trees can be useful in inhalations and washes.

Parts used: Leaves, essential oil

Actions: Antiseptic, antiviral, antifungal, antispasmodic, stimulant, febrifuge, hypoglycaemic

Used in: Steam inhalations, chest rubs, infusions, tinctures, capsules/tablets

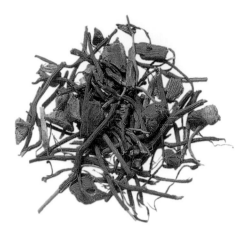

Hemp agrimony *Eupatorium cannabium*

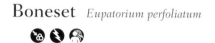

A popular medieval wound herb, the leaves of hemp agrimony were once commonly wrapped around bread to prevent mould from forming. The herb is now known to be an immune stimulant, increasing resistance to viral infections.

Parts used: Root, aerial parts

Actions: Febrifuge, diuretic, antiscorbutic, laxative, tonic, bile stimulant, expectorant, diaphoretic, antirheumatic, immune stimulant

Used in: Infusions, decoctions, capsules, tinctures

Cautions: High doses may cause nausea and the fresh herb can be purgative

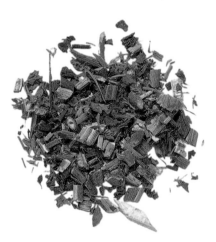

Boneset *Eupatorium perfoliatum*

Boneset is so called from its traditional use in North America as a remedy for flu-type fevers with their associated aches and pains. The settlers soon adopted the herb as a cure-all and it reached Europe in the 19th century.

Parts used: Aerial parts

Actions: Immune stimulant, diaphoretic, peripheral vasodilator, laxative, bile stimulant

Used in: Infusions, tinctures

Eyebright *Euphrasia officinalis*

A tiny, semi-parasitic plant growing in grassy meadows, eyebright has been used as a remedy for eye problems (*see* Conjunctivitis *and* Herbal eyebaths, *pages* 135, 136) since at least the 14th century. It can be extremely effective for relieving the more irritant symptoms of hay fever and is an effective anticatarrhal for catarrh and sinusitis (*see pages* 96, 97).

Parts used: Aerial parts

Actions: Anti-inflammatory, antihistamine, anticatarrhal, astringent

Used in: Infusions, capsules, tincture, eyebaths

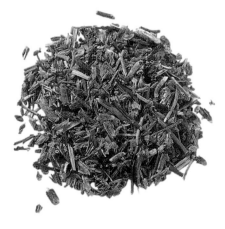

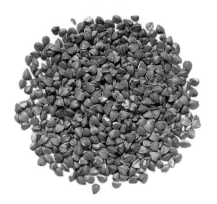

Buckwheat *Fagopyrum esculentum*

Buckwheat was brought to Europe by the Crusaders as a cereal crop and is still used for crêpes in Brittany and polenta in Italy. It is rich in rutin, which strengthens blood vessels (*see* Poor circulation, *page* 91, Varicose veins, *page* 92), lowers blood pressure and controls bleeding.

Parts used: Flowers, leaves, seeds (used in cooking)

Actions: Vein tonic and restorative, hypotensive, peripheral vasodilator, anticoagulant

Used in: Infusions, capsules

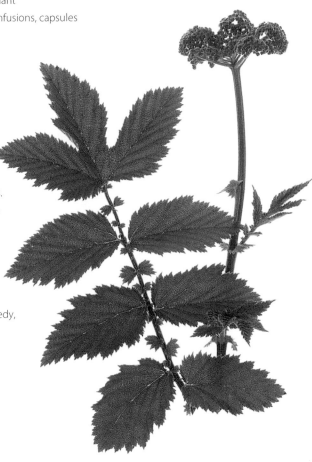

Meadowsweet *Filipendula ulmaria*

Meadowsweet's old botanical name, *Spiraea ulmaria*, gave its name to the drug aspirin which was patented by Bayer in the 1890s. The herb was an original source of salicylate compounds, which are similar in action to those now synthesized in the familiar drug. It is used internally for gastritis (*see page* 120) and indigestion and heartburn (*see page* 123) as well as easing arthritic and rheumatic aches and pains (*see page* 131).

Parts used: Aerial parts, leaves

Actions: Anti-inflammatory, antirheumatic, soothing digestive remedy, diuretic, diaphoretic, antacid, astringent

Used in: Tinctures, infusions, powders, compresses, eyebaths

Caution: Meadowsweet is best avoided by those sensitive to salicylates and aspirin

Fennel -*Foeniculum vulgare*

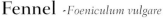

Familiar as a vegetable and culinary herb, fennel is also a valuable medicinal plant. It is largely used for indigestion (*see page* 121), flatulence and colic (*see page* 149), but it will also help to increase milk flow in nursing mothers and can be used as a mouthwash and gargle for gum disease and sore throats.

Parts used: Seeds, essential oil, aerial parts, root

Actions: Carminative, circulatory stimulant, anti-inflammatory, stimulates milk flow, mild expectorant, diuretic

Used in: Infusions, decoctions, tinctures, gargles and mouthwashes, massage rubs

Caution: Avoid high doses in pregnancy

Lian Qiao (Forsythia) *Forsythia suspensa*

Widely cultivated as a garden shrub, forsythia berries are an important Chinese herb for combating all types of infection – from colds and flu to mumps and glandular problems.

Parts used: Fruits

Actions: Antibacterial, febrifuge, diuretic, bitter digestive stimulant, antiemetic

Used in: Decoctions, tinctures

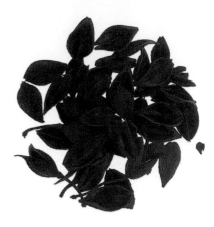

Bladderwrack *Fucus vesiculosis*

The seaweed, bladderwrack, is a salty, tonic herb, rich in iodine and trace metals and a good source of essential nutrients. The iodine content stimulates the thyroid and thus speeds up body metabolism – hence bladderwrack's reputation as a slimming aid. Infused bladderwrack oil can be used externally for rheumatic and arthritic problems.

Parts used: Whole plant (thalli)

Actions: Metabolic stimulant, nutritive, thyroid tonic, antirheumatic, anti-inflammatory

Used in: Capsules/tablets, tinctures, infused oils, infusions

Cautions: Bladderwrack will concentrate toxic waste metals such as cadmium and strontium which pollute our oceans and should not be collected in contaminated areas

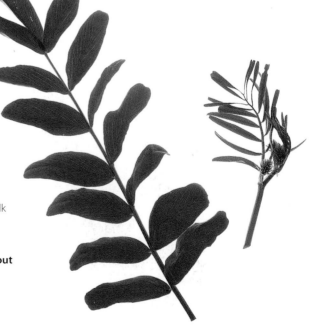

Goat's rue *Galega officinalis*

Once a favourite treatment for plague, goat's rue is now largely used in late-onset diabetes (*see page* 139) to normalize blood sugar levels. It is also a milk stimulant and will reputedly increase breast size.

Parts used: Leaves

Actions: Antidiabetic, hypoglycaemic, diuretic, diaphoretic, increases milk flow

Used in: Infusions, tinctures, capsules

Caution: Should not be taken by insulin-dependent diabetics without professional supervision

Cleavers *Galium aparine*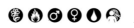

Usually dismissed as a weed, cleavers can be found scrambling through shrubs in most suburban gardens. It is an important lymphatic cleanser that was once used to feed domestic geese, hence its country name, 'goosegrass'.

Parts used: Aerial parts
Actions: Diuretic, lymphatic cleanser, mild astringent
Used in: Infusions, juices, tinctures, creams

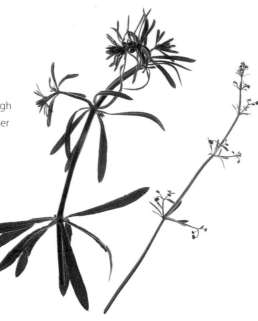

Reishi *Ganoderma lucidem*

The reishi mushroom was highly regarded by the ancient Chinese Taoists as a spiritual tonic and one which could enhance longevity. The herb is now known to stimulate the immune system, making it valuable for recurrent infections (*see page* 127) and debility. It has been used for chronic fatigue syndrome (*see page* 104) and AIDS.

Part used: Fruiting body
Actions: Hypotensive, hypoglycaemic, antiviral, immune stimulant, expectorant, antitussive, antihistamine, antitumour
Used in: Tinctures, powders, capsules

Ginkgo *Ginkgo biloba*

Ginkgo has been grown in many botanical gardens as an ornamental since 1727. It is a deciduous conifer – a rare fossil survivor. Recent research has demonstrated that it will significantly improve cerebral circulation and it is now used for a wide range of blood disorders. In traditional Chinese medicine it is recommended for asthma and urinary problems.

Parts used: Leaves, seeds (in traditional Chinese medicine)
Actions: *Leaves:* Vasodilator, circulatory stimulant, anti-inflammatory; *Seeds:* Astringent, antifungal, antibacterial
Used in: Tablets/capsules, tinctures, infusions, decoctions, fluid extracts

Ground ivy *Glechoma hederacea*

Used in brewing in the 16th century, hence its common name, alehoof, ground ivy is helpful for sinus (*see page* 97) and ear problems as well as for soothing gastritis and cystitis (*see page* 114). Lotions containing ground ivy can be used externally for piles and throat inflammations.

Parts used: Aerial parts

Actions: Anticatarrhal, astringent, expectorant, diuretic

Used in: Infusions, tinctures, capsules

Liquorice *Glycyrrhiza glabra*

Liquorice contains glycyrrhizin, which is 50 times sweeter than sucrose and encourages production of hormones like hydrocortisone. It is soothing for the digestive tract, hence its traditional use in treating gastric ulcers, and is a popular laxative for constipation (*see page* 120).

Part used: Root

Actions: Anti-inflammatory, antiarthritic, tonic stimulant for adrenal cortex, hypoglycaemic, soothing for gastric mucosa, possibly antiallergenic, antipyretic, expectorant, laxative

Used in: Tinctures, fluid extracts, decoctions, dried juice sticks, powders

Cautions: Excessive liquorice can cause fluid retention and increase blood pressure, therefore avoid if you have hypertension. Do not use if taking digoxin-based drugs

Witch hazel *Hamamelis virginiana*

Distilled witch hazel is a familiar first aid remedy for bruises, sprains, cuts, and grazes. It is commonly used to ease varicose veins and piles, applied to spots and blemishes, and valuable for all sorts of minor injuries. Witch hazel is used internally for diarrhoea, colitis, heavy periods, and haemorrhage.

Parts used: Leaves, branches, bark

Actions: Astringent, stops bleeding

Used in: Distillates, tinctures, infusions

Devil's claw *Harpagophytum procumbens*

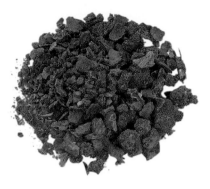

Devil's claw grows in the Kalahari Desert in South Africa and takes its name from the shape of its seed pods. It was reputedly introduced into Western medicine by a South African farmer who noticed bushmen using it in decoctions for a number of ills – notably digestive upsets and rheumatism. It is now popular for arthritis (*see page* 131).

Part used: Tuberous root

Actions: Anti-inflammatory, analgesic, digestive stimulant, liver tonic, bile stimulant, diuretic, stimulant

Used in: Decoctions, capsules/tablets, tinctures, creams, massage rubs

Caution: Devil's claw is believed to stimulate uterine contractions and should be avoided in pregnancy

Hops *Humulus lupulus*

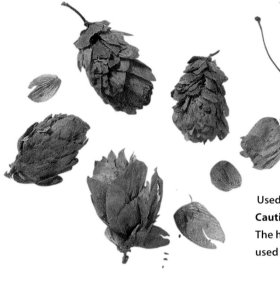

Hops have been used in brewing in Germany since the 11th century, although they were not introduced to England until the 16th century when contemporary herbalists condemned them as 'encouraging melancholy'. They are also male anaphrodisiacs: excessive consumption of beer can lead to a loss of libido. Hops are a bitter digestive stimulant and are useful for stress, irritability and insomnia (*see page* 104).

Parts used: Strobiles (female flowers)

Actions: Sedative, anaphrodisiac, restoring tonic for the nervous system, bitter digestive stimulant, diuretic

Used in: Infusions, tinctures, herb pillows, capsules, compresses

Cautions: Hops should not be taken by those suffering from depression. The hormonal content may disrupt the normal menstrual cycle when used regularly

Golden seal *Hydrastis canadensis*

Golden seal was once used by the Cherokee for digestive problems and to make an insect-repellent ointment. The root has a bitter taste and acts as a digestive stimulant but the plant will also combat infections and is useful for catarrh (*see page* 96) and hay fever (*see page* 97). It can ease hot flushes at the menopause (*see page* 115).

Part used: Rhizome

Actions: Astringent, tonic, anti-inflammatory, bitter, digestive and bile stimulant, anticatarrhal, laxative, healing to gastric mucosa, possibly hypertensive, uterine stimulant

Used in: Tinctures, capsules, gargles, douches

Cautions: Avoid in pregnancy and if you have high blood pressure

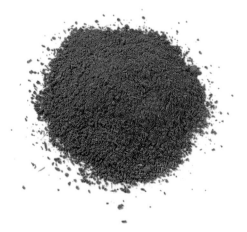

St John's wort   *Hypericum perforatum*

Although a traditional wound herb and pain remedy, St John's wort is now becoming better known as an antidepressant (*see page* 101) and is widely prescribed by German doctors. It has also been used in AIDS treatments, and is a valuable external remedy for minor burns and grazes (*see pages* 114, 115).

Parts used: Flowering tops

Actions: Astringent, analgesic, anti-inflammatory, sedative, restoring tonic for the nervous system, antidepressant, antispasmodic, antiviral

Used in: Infused oils, infusions, tinctures, creams, capsules/tablets

Caution: Prolonged use may increase the photosensitivity of the skin

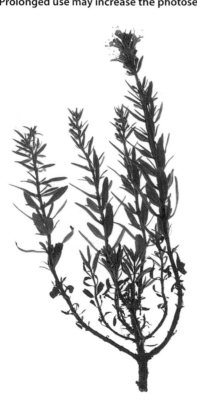

Hyssop   *Hyssopus officinale*

Like other members of the mint family, hyssop is a bitter digestive tonic and useful in cooking. However, its main medicinal application is for upper respiratory tract infections, congestion, coughs (*see page* 96) and feverish chills. As a digestive remedy it can be useful for flatulence and colic and is quite safe to use with children. The essential oil is also mildly sedative and can be added to relaxing baths.

Parts used: Aerial parts, essential oil

Actions: Expectorant, carminative, peripheral vasodilator, diaphoretic, anticatarrhal, topically anti-inflammatory, antiviral (*Herpes simplex*)

Used in: Infusions, tinctures, syrups, massage rubs, baths

Caution: Excessive use of the essential oil may cause convulsions

Elecampane   *Inula helenium*

In the 8th century, elecampane was regarded as a remedy for 'elf-shot' and 'evil eye'. Today, it is an important expectorant and lung tonic (*see* Asthma *and* Bronchitis, *page* 95), mainly used in cough and catarrh remedies. It is a useful restorative for the debility that can follow bouts of influenza. Although the root is used in Western herbalism, the Chinese use the flowers of a related species in very similar ways.

Parts used: Root, flowers

Actions: Tonic, stimulating expectorant, diaphoretic, antibacterial, antifungal, antiparasitic

Used in: Decoctions, tinctures, syrups

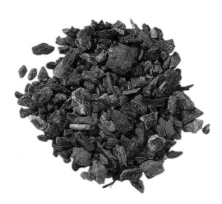

White deadnettle *Lamium album*

Mainly used for menstrual and urinary disorders: deadnettle tea can be helpful for cystitis (*see page* 114) and in prostatitis (*see page* 108) and it can be useful to speed recovery after surgery for enlarged prostate. It can also be taken for heavy periods (*see page* 112) and used as a douche for vaginal discharges. Deadnettle creams and ointments can be used externally on cuts, grazes and minor burns.

Parts used: Aerial parts collected while flowering

Actions: Anti-inflammatory, antispasmodic, astringent, diuretic, expectorant, menstrual regulator, styptic, wound herb

Used in: Infusions, tinctures, creams

Lavender

Lavandula angustifolia

A valuable herb for numerous health problems, including headaches (*see page* 134), digestive upsets and nervous problems.

Parts used: Flowers, essential oil

Actions: Antiseptic, antibacterial, antidepressant, carminative, relaxant, antispasmodic, circulatory stimulant, tonic for the nervous system, analgesic, bile stimulant

Used in: Infusions, tinctures, massage rubs

Caution: Avoid high doses in pregnancy

Motherwort *Leonurus cardiaca*

Used as a heart tonic, motherwort takes its name from its traditional use – calming anxiety in childbirth. It may also help prevent thrombosis, and is popular for treating menopausal upsets (*see page* 115) and PMT.

Parts used: Aerial parts

Actions: Uterine stimulant, relaxant, cardiac tonic, carminative

Used in: Infusions, tinctures, syrups, douches

Caution: Avoid in pregnancy, except in labour, as it is a uterine stimulant

Bugleweed *Lycopus virginicus* ⬤

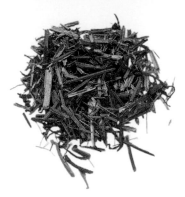

Bugleweed, also known as gypsywort, is largely used to relieve the symptoms of an overactive thyroid gland, especially rapid heartbeat and palpitations. It can be helpful for low blood sugar levels and has a traditional use in parts of Europe as a contraceptive.

Parts used: Aerial parts

Actions: Sedative, astringent, tonic, vasoconstrictor, antitussive, hyperglycaemic, stops bleeding

Used in: Infusions, tinctures

Caution: Avoid in pregnancy

White horehound *Marrubium vulgare*
⬤⬤⬤

Horehound candy was once widely available from confectioners and chemists as a remedy for coughs and the herb is still used for bronchitis, colds and catarrh. It is a good liver stimulant and can be used externally for grazes and skin rashes although it is more often regarded as an internal remedy.

Part used: Leaves

Actions: Stimulating expectorant, bitter digestive tonic, antispasmodic, sedative, wound herb, diuretic

Used in: Infusions, syrups, tinctures, lozenges, creams, ointments

Chamomile *Matricaria recutita*
⬤⬤⬤⬤⬤⬤⬤⬤⬤

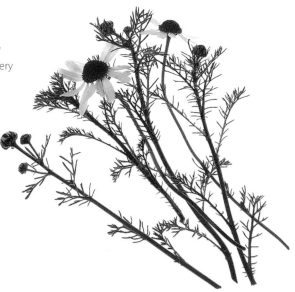

Both German chamomile and its relative Roman chamomile (*Chamaemelum nobile*) are among the most widely used medicinal herbs. Their actions are very similar; Roman chamomile has a slightly more bitter taste and German chamomile is slightly more anti-inflammatory and analgesic. The flowers are popular in tisanes and as a hair rinse for fair hair. They are also used in homeopathic remedies for teething and colic (*see page* 149). Chamomile flowers will produce a deep blue essential oil on steam distillation, which is very relaxing and useful in skin care.

Part used: Flowers, essential oil

Actions: Anti-inflammatory, antispasmodic, bitter, sedative, carminative, antiemetic, antiallergenic

Used in: Infusions, steam inhalations, tinctures, creams, baths, massage rubs, ointments

Caution: The fresh plant can cause contact dermatitis in sensitive individuals

Tea tree *Melaleuca alternifolia*

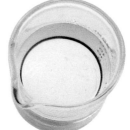

European interest in the Australian tea tree dates back to the 1920s when the strong antibacterial action of its oil was first investigated in France. Extracts were used in traditional Aboriginal medicine, and in the past few years a thriving tea tree industry has grown up which has led to a number of highly adulterated oils appearing on the market. True tea tree oil is one of the few which does not usually irritate mucous membranes and it can be used neat on the skin.

Part used: Essential oil

Actions: Antiseptic, antibacterial, antifungal, antiviral, immune stimulant, antiparasitic

Used in: Creams, lotions, ointments, pessaries, shampoos

Melilot *Melilotus officinale* ♡

Melilot smells of new mown hay – due to the coumarins it contains which account for much of its antithrombotic action. It is useful for easing the pain and eczema associated with varicose veins (*see page* 92) and can also be helpful for facial neuralgia (*see page* 104) and rheumatic pains or in eyebaths for conjunctivitis.

Parts used: Aerial parts

Actions: Anticoagulant, antithrombotic, antispasmodic, anti-inflammatory, diuretic, expectorant, sedative, styptic, mild analgesic

Used in: Infusions, tinctures, ointments, creams, compresses, powders, eyebaths

Caution: Do not take melilot if using anticoagulant drugs, such as warfarin

Lemon balm *Melissa officinalis*

Lemon balm was associated by the ancient Greeks with bees and the healing power of honey – hence its botanical name, from the Latin for honey (*mel*). It is a gentle herb useful for treating nervous tummy upsets in children but it is also potent enough to help with depression, anxiety and tension headaches. Lemon balm creams can be used externally on insect bites (*see page* 147), sores and slow-healing wounds.

Parts used: Aerial parts, essential oil (known as melissa oil)

Actions: Sedative, antidepressant, digestive stimulant, peripheral vasodilator, diaphoretic, relaxing restorative for the nervous system, antiviral, antibacterial

Used in: Infusions, tinctures, creams, baths, insect-repellent sprays

Peppermint *Mentha X piperita*

Peppermint is a cross between spearmint and watermint and its characteristic smell is due to a high menthol content. Numerous varieties have been grown over the years: perhaps the most famous was Mitcham mint, a black peppermint which once formed an important cash crop in what are now London's southern suburbs. The herb is largely used to relieve flatulence (*see page* 123), bloating and colic, although it is also useful for catarrh and travel sickness.

Parts used: Aerial parts, essential oil

Actions: Antispasmodic, digestive tonic, antiemetic, carminative, peripheral vasodilator, diaphoretic, bile stimulant, analgesic

Used in: Infusions, tinctures, lotions, capsules, steam inhalations, compresses, massage rubs

Cautions: Avoid prolonged or excessive use as it can irritate the mucous membranes. Do not use the herb with children under four or the oil on those under ten years old

Nutmeg *Myristica fragrans*

Despite its familiarity as a kitchen seasoning, nutmeg is actually quite a potent hallucinogen and soporific: cases of delirium resulting from over-consumption were reported as early as 1576. In low doses it is ideal for digestive problems such as nausea, abdominal bloating, indigestion and colic.

Parts used: Seed kernel (nutmeg), aril (mace), essential oil

Actions: Carminative, digestive stimulant, antispasmodic, antiemetic, appetite stimulant, anti-inflammatory

Used in: Powders, ointments, decoctions, capsules, massage rub

Cautions: Large doses – 5 g or more in a single dose – can produce convulsions. Avoid in pregnancy

Catmint *Nepeta cataria*

Catmint is a favourite with cats who will roll in ecstasy in a bed of the plant. It is a gentle herb ideal for children and suitable for colic (*see page* 149), feverish chills and hyperactivity. Like other members of the mint family it will also ease the symptoms of indigestion, but unlike peppermint it does not contain irritant menthol. (The ornamental cultivar, shown here, is less therapeutic than its white-blossomed counterpart.)

Parts used: Aerial parts

Actions: Antispasmodic, diaphoretic, carminative, gentle nerve relaxant, antidiarrhoeal, increases menstrual flow

Used in: Infusions, compresses, ointments, lotions, rubs

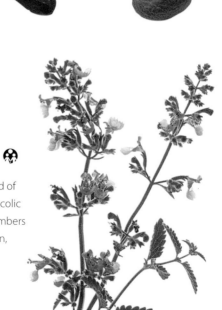

Basil *Ocimum basilicum*

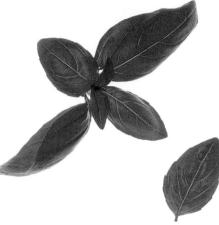

Familiar in Europe as a culinary herb, basil is regarded in India as a potent tonic – sacred to Vishnu and Krishna and capable of 'opening the heart and mind'. More prosaically, Western herbalism recommends it for digestive upsets, to clear intestinal parasites and to improve digestion. The oil can be used as a nerve tonic, antidepressant (*see page* 101) and digestive remedy.

Parts used: Leaves, essential oil

Actions: Antidepressant, antiseptic, stimulates the adrenal cortex, antiemetic, tonic, carminative, febrifuge, expectorant

Used in: Infusions, decoctions, baths, juices, fresh leaves, syrups, inhalations, powders, massage rubs

Caution: Do not use basil oil in pregnancy

Evening primrose

Oenetheris biennis

Evening primrose is a North American plant traditionally used in infusions for asthma and digestive disorders. Its seeds are rich in the essential fatty acid gamma-linolenic acid (GLA) – a precursor of prostaglandin E_1 which inhibits abnormal cell proliferation. A lack of GLA has been associated with systemic rheumatic and skin disorders. The oil is also reputed to ease menstrual and menopausal problems, strengthen the circulatory system and boost the immune system.

Parts used: Seed oil

Actions: Anti-eczema, demulcent, antithrombotic

Used in: Capsules, creams

Caution: Do not take the oil if suffering from epilepsy

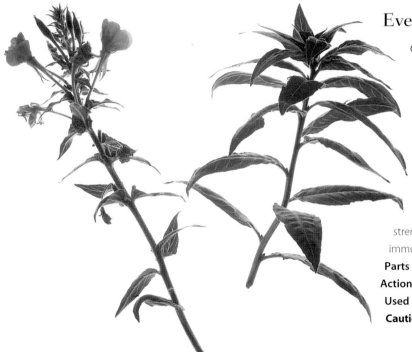

Ginseng *Panax ginseng*

Ginseng has been used in China for more than 5000 years and is believed to strengthen the body's vital energy (*Qi*). The plant is rich in steroidal compounds which are very similar to human sex hormones, hence its reputation as an aphrodisiac. It is, however, a rather more all-round tonic, helping the body adapt to stressful situations; it is especially valuable for the elderly and to strengthen the lungs. As a general tonic it is ideally taken for a month in late autumn when the weather is changing from hot summer to cold winter, when the body needs to adapt to the new environment.

Parts used: Root, tablets, tonic wine, decoction

Actions: Tonic, stimulant, hypoglycaemic, reduces cholesterol levels, immune stimulant

Used in: Capsules

Cautions: Do not take for more than four weeks without a break. Avoid taking with caffeine and in pregnancy

Passion flower *Passiflora incarnata*

Passion flower takes its name from the religious symbolism of its flowers rather than any therapeutic effects. It was traditionally used by Native Americans as a tonic and remedy for epilepsy. Today it is regarded as an effective but gentle sedative largely used for insomnia (*see page* 104).

Parts used: Aerial parts

Actions: Sedative, antispasmodic, vasodilator, analgesic, tranquillizer

Used in: Infusions, tinctures, capsules

Cautions: Avoid high doses in pregnancy. May cause drowsiness

Parsley *Petroselinum crispum*

Although more familiar as a garnish, parsley is also a valuable medicinal herb; it is also a good source of vitamins and minerals – a useful addition to the diet in anaemia (*see page* 92). It is often used as a diuretic for premenstrual fluid retention and is a cleansing remedy in rheumatism. Chewing fresh parsley reputedly reduces the lingering smell of garlic.

Parts used: Leaves, roots, seeds

Actions: Antispasmodic, antirheumatic, diuretic, carminative, expectorant, tonic, antimicrobial, nutrient

Used in: Infusions, juices, tinctures, capsules, fresh leaves

Caution: Avoid therapeutic doses in pregnancy

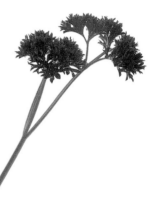

Ribwort plantain *Plantago lanceolata*

Ribwort plantain has long pointed leaves and will grow to around 30-40 cm/12–16 in – quite unlike its familiar relative common plantain (*see page* 71). It is an effective anticatarrhal largely used for colds and hay fever. It also concentrates minerals and trace elements from the soil in its leaves so it is very healing and supportive for the immune system.

Parts used: Leaves

Actions: Relaxing expectorant, tonifying to mucous membranes, anticatarrhal, antispasmodic

Used in: Infusions, tinctures, capsules

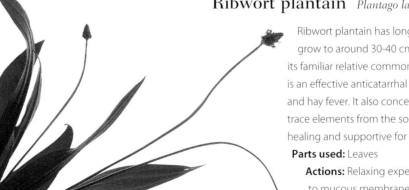

Common plantain

Plantago major

Common plantain can be used fresh as a
wound herb or for insect stings. The plant is very
widespread – it even became known as 'white
man's foot' in North America because it spread
with the settlers. It is a very versatile herb and can
be used for gastric inflammations, cystitis, diarrhoea, respiratory
problems and catarrh. Ointments containing the herb can be used
for slow-healing wounds, burns and piles (*see page* 92).

Parts used: Leaves

Actions: Antibacterial, antiallergenic, blood and lymphatic tonic, styptic, diuretic,
expectorant, demulcent, astringent

Used in: Infusions, capsules, tinctures, compresses, juices, ointments, fresh leaves

Ispaghula   *Plantago psyllium; P. ovata*

Ispaghula is widely used as a bulking laxative: the seeds swell when moistened to form
a glutinous mass which encourages peristalsis (muscular contraction of the
alimentary tract during digestion) and lubricates the bowel. Although primarily
used for constipation (*see page* 120), the resulting bulky mass can help to soothe
diarrhoea and is sometimes recommended in irritable bowel syndrome.

Parts used: Seeds, husks

Actions: Demulcent, bulk laxative, antidiarrhoeal

Used in: Macerations, poultices, capsules

**Caution: Always take capsules or dried ispaghula with
plenty of water**

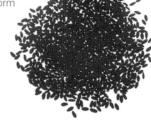

Bistort   *Polygonum bistorta*

Bistort is believed to be the Saxon *atterlothe* – one of
the nine great healing herbs which the god Woden
gave to the world. It is an extremely astringent plant
largely used for bleeding – both internal and external –
and for diarrhoea (*see page* 121). A little powdered root
in the nostrils is a useful standby for nosebleeds
(*see page* 98).

Parts used: Root and rhizome

Actions: Astringent, antidiarrhoeal, anti-inflammatory,
anticatarrhal, demulcent, styptic

Used in: Decoctions, tinctures, powders, mouthwashes and gargles,
ointments

He Shou Wu (Flowery knotweed)

Polygonum multiflorum ♂ ♀

He Shou Wu – also known as *Fo Ti* in Cantonese – is one of the most popular Chinese tonic herbs. It is believed to restore liver and kidney *Qi* and is often included in menopausal remedies where the Chinese believe this sort of energy to be particularly weak. The Chinese also use it to combat premature ageing and to restore the colour to greying hair.

Part used: Root

Actions: Sedative, blood tonic, energy tonic

Used in: Decoctions, tinctures, powders, capsules, tonic wines

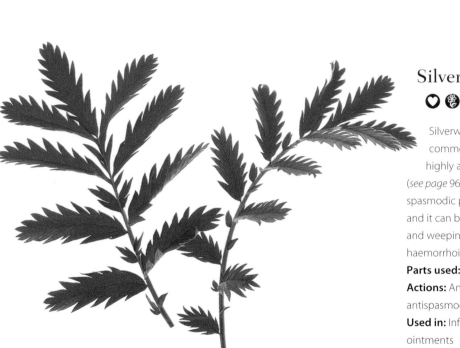

Silverweed *Potentilla anserina*
♡ ✿

Silverweed is a decorative, low growing plant commonly cultivated as a garden flower. It is highly astringent and useful to combat catarrh (*see page* 96) and as a wound herb. It also eases spasmodic pain, such as period cramps and colic, and it can be used externally as a wash for sores and weeping eczema or as an ointment for haemorrhoids.

Parts used: Leaves, flowers

Actions: Anti-inflammatory, astringent, antispasmodic, diuretic, styptic

Used in: Infusions, tinctures, compresses, gargles, ointments

Cowslip *Primula veris* ✿ 🔥

Cowslip roots are rich in saponins, making the plant a potent expectorant for harsh, difficult coughs and sticky mucous that is difficult to shift. The root also contains salicylates and has been used for arthritis. The flowers contain neither of these chemicals and are mainly used as a relaxing nervine for insomnia (*see page* 104) and tension.

Parts used: Root, flowers

Actions: *Root:* Stimulating expectorant, antispasmodic, anti-inflammatory, astringent; *Flowers:* Sedative nervine

Used in: Infusions, decoctions, tinctures

Cautions: Avoid in pregnancy or in cases of salicylate allergy

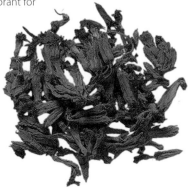

Self-heal (*Xu Ku Cao*) *Prunella vulgaris*

Self-heal – as the name implies – is a traditional European wound herb widely used to stop bleeding and ease inflammations. The Chinese use the flower spikes quite differently – as a cooling remedy for the liver, and for fevers, hyperactivity, dizziness and vertigo. Modern research has confirmed that it can reduce high blood pressure.

Parts used: Leaves, flower spikes

Actions: *Leaves/aerial parts:* Antibacterial, hypotensive, diuretic, astringent, wound herb; *Spikes:* Liver stimulant

Used in: Tinctures, infusions, decoctions, poultices, ointments, eyebaths, mouthwashes and gargles

Da Huang (Chinese rhubarb)

Rheum palmatum

The Chinese name for rhubarb root means 'big yellow' and refers to its rich colour. The medicinal plant is different from the edible variety, which was hybridized in the 19th century. Rhubarb root is used for chronic constipation (*see page* 120) and for liver and gall bladder problems.

Part used: Root

Actions: Laxative, digestive remedy, astringent

Used in: Decoctions, tinctures

Caution: Avoid rhubarb root in pregnancy or during lactation

Rose *Rosa* spp

The rose is probably one of the West's most neglected medicinal herbs, although until the 1930s it was regularly prescribed for sore throats and diarrhoea. Rosehips are still valued as an important source of vitamin C and rose oil is used for skin and emotional problems. Various varieties of rose are used in Chinese medicine as tonics, and for liver and menstrual disorders.

Parts used: Petals, rosehips, essential oil

Actions: Antidepressant, antispasmodic, aphrodisiac, astringent, sedative, digestive stimulant, bile stimulant, cleansing, expectorant, antibacterial, antiviral, antiseptic

Used in: Infusions, tinctures, syrups, decoctions, creams, lotions, massage rubs, gargles and mouthwashes

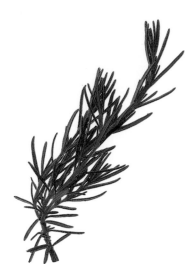

Rosemary *Rosmarinus officinalis*

Rosemary is a stimulating tonic herb – very warming and useful for temporary fatigue and overwork. It makes a pleasant tea. The herb also stimulates circulation and can relieve headaches and migraine (*see page* 135), indigestion and the cold feelings from poor circulation. The oil is also a valuable remedy for arthritis, rheumatism, and muscular aches and pains. It is reputed to darken greying hair, makes a good rinse for auburn hair and helps clear dandruff.

Parts used: Leaves, essential oil

Actions: *Leaves/aerial parts:* Astringent, digestive remedy, nervine, carminative, antiseptic, diuretic, diaphoretic, antidepressant, circulatory stimulant, antispasmodic, restorative tonic for the nervous system, bile stimulant, cardiac tonic; *Essential oil:* Topically rubefacient, analgesic, antirheumatic

Used in: Tinctures, infusions, infused oils, compresses, shampoos, massage rubs

Raspberry *Rubus idaeus*

Raspberry leaf is best known for its tonifying effect on the uterus and its use as a preparative for childbirth (*see page* 115). It is generally taken for six to eight weeks before the confinement and during labour to help strengthen the womb. It is also used as a gargle for sore throats (*see page* 97), and may be taken for diarrhoea.

Parts used: Leaves, fruit

Actions: Astringent, birth preparative, stimulant, digestive remedy, tonic, diuretic, laxative

Used in: Infusions, tinctures, gargles, vinegars

Caution: Avoid high doses of the leaves during the first six months of pregnancy

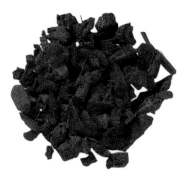

Yellow dock *Rumex crispus*

Yellow dock is a cleansing herb suitable for chronic skin problems, and also for arthritic complaints (*see page* 131). It is also a laxative but is rather gentler than strong purgatives like rhubarb.

Part used: Root

Actions: Laxative, bile stimulant, cleansing

Used in: Decoctions, tinctures

Caution: Avoid high doses in pregnancy and during lactation

White willow   *Salix alba*

The *Salix* genus gives its name to salicylates – the group of anti-inflammatory and analgesic compounds familiar in aspirin and present in significant amounts in the bark and leaves of the white willow. The plant, like aspirin, is used for relieving pain and reducing fevers, and is helpful for rheumatism, gout (*see page* 133), arthritis, feverish chills and headaches.

Part used: Bark

Actions: Antirheumatic, anti-inflammatory, antipyretic, antihidrotic, analgesic, antiseptic, astringent, bitter digestive tonic

Used in: Tinctures, fluid extracts, decoctions, capsules/tablets

Caution: Avoid in salicylate allergy

Sage   *Salvia officinalis*

Useful for menopausal problems (*see page* 115), minor infections and gum inflammations, sage ointment is also used in parts of Europe for minor cuts and insect bites.

Parts used: Leaves, essential oil

Actions: *Leaves:* Carminative, antispasmodic, astringent and healing to mucosa, antiseptic, peripheral vasodilator, suppresses perspiration, reduces salivation and lactation, uterine stimulant, systemically antibiotic, hypoglycaemic, bile stimulant; *Essential oil:* Antiseptic, antispasmodic, astringent, hypertensive, stimulant, stimulates menstruation, antioxidant

Used in: Infusions, tinctures, ointments, fresh leaves, massage rubs, compresses, mouthwashes and gargles, hair rinses

Cautions: Avoid high doses in pregnancy or if epileptic

Elder   *Sambucus nigra*

Once regarded as a complete medicine chest, today only the flowers are widely used, although berry juice is still available. The flowers strengthen the mucous membranes of the upper respiratory tract and increase resistance to irritant allergens.

Parts used: Flowers, berries, stem bark, root, leaves

Actions: *Flowers:* Expectorant, anticatarrhal, circulatory stimulant, diaphoretic, diuretic; Locally – Anti-inflammatory. *Berries:* Diaphoretic, diuretic, laxative. *Bark:* Internally – Strong purgative, emetic (in large doses), diuretic; Externally – Softening. *Leaves:* Externally – softening, wound healing; Internally – purgative, expectorant, diuretic, diaphoretic. *Root:* Violent emetic and purgative (not used nowadays)

Used in: Infusions, tinctures, creams, eyebaths, gargles and mouthwashes, ointments, syrups, decoctions

Caution: Avoid high doses of elder bark in pregnancy

Sandalwood *Santalum alba*

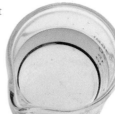

Sandalwood is important in Ayurvedic medicine as a cooling herb that stimulates the mind and improves digestive energy. In aromatherapy the oil is regarded as relaxing and antidepressant; it is used for urinary problems, nervous disorders and chest complaints and can be added to bath water to encourage restful sleep.

Parts used: Wood, essential oil

Actions: Antiseptic, antibacterial, urinary antiseptic, carminative, relaxing, diuretic, antispasmodic

Used in: Massage rubs, baths, pastes

Skullcap *Scutellaria lateriflora*

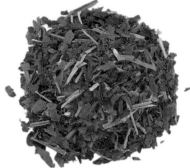

The variety of skullcap most widely used in medicine today originated in Virginia in the USA and was introduced into Europe in the 18th century as a treatment for rabies – hence the alternative name of 'mad dog'. Today, it is mainly used as a relaxing sedative for stress and anxiety, although in the past it was recommended for jaundice, urinary tract infections, haemorrhage and threatened miscarriage.

Parts used: Aerial parts

Actions: Relaxing and restorative nervine, antispasmodic, bitter

Used in: Infusions, tinctures, capsules

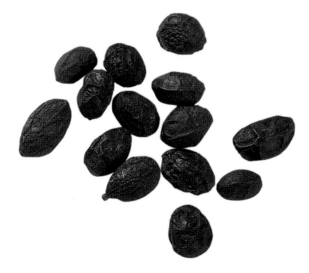

Saw palmetto *Serenoa repens*

Saw palmetto berries originated in the south-eastern states of the USA and were highly valued for their tonic effect, as a strengthening remedy in debility and for cystitis and prostate problems. Modern research has shown that the herb prevents the conversion of the male hormone testosterone into dihydrotestosterone which is believed to be responsible for benign prostate enlargement.

Parts used: Berries

Actions: Tonic, diuretic, sedative, urinary antiseptic, tonic, endocrine stimulant, hormonal action

Used in: Decoctions, tinctures, capsules

Milk thistle *Silybum marianum*

Today, milk thistle is usually regarded as a protective remedy for the liver (*see* Liver problems, *page* 124). It contains silymarin, which has been shown to prevent toxic chemicals from damaging the liver and has also been successfully used for cirrhosis of the liver and hepatitis. Formerly the plant was used to encourage milk flow in nursing mothers – hence its name.

Parts used: Seeds

Actions: Bitter tonic, protects the liver, bile stimulant, increases milk flow, antidepressant, antiviral

Used in: Infusions, tinctures, capsules

Golden rod

Solidago vigaurea

Today, golden rod is largely used as a diuretic and urinary antiseptic for treating kidney and bladder problems, but it is also effective for catarrh and coughs and can be helpful for tonsillitis and sore throats. It is used externally for sores and ulcers.

Parts used: Leaves and flowers

Actions: Anticatarrhal, anti-inflammatory, antiseptic, diuretic, diaphoretic

Used in: Infusions, tinctures, compresses, gargles

Wood betony *Stachys officinalis*

Although held in high regard by the Anglo-Saxons, who had some 29 medicinal uses for the plant, wood betony has now largely fallen out of fashion. However, it is an excellent remedy for headaches and nervous upsets, is useful for liver and respiratory disorders, and it also makes a pleasant tisane for everyday drinking.

Parts used: Aerial parts

Actions: Sedative, bitter digestive remedy, nervine, circulatory tonic particularly for cerebral circulation, astringent

Used in: Infusions, tinctures, poultices, mouthwashes and gargles, tonic wines

Caution: Avoid in pregnancy except during labour

Chickweed *Stellaria media*

As the name implies, chickweed has long been used for feeding domestic fowl. It is an extremely common garden weed and makes a popular, soothing cream for irritant skin rashes and eczema, and is a good first aid treatment for burns, boils and drawing splinters. It was once regarded as a significant source of vitamin C, with sprigs added to salads or cooked as a vegetable.

Parts used: Aerial parts

Actions: Astringent, antirheumatic, wound herb, demulcent

Used in: Tinctures, infusions, infused oils, creams, ointments

Comfrey *Symphytum officinalis*

Comfrey has undergone a chequered history in recent years: alternatively acclaimed as a panacea and banned as a health hazard. It is restricted in many countries because it contains pyrrolizidine alkaloids (known carcinogens), although it is debatable how much of these toxic chemicals are actually present in comfrey tinctures, teas, and ointment. As a precaution it is best confined to external remedies for home use, and is excellent for treating bruises, sprains and even fractures. It is used internally by herbalists for coughs, stomach ulceration and digestive upsets.

Parts used: Root, leaves

Actions: Cell proliferator, astringent, demulcent, wound herb, expectorant

Used in: Ointments, infused oils, creams, washes, compresses, poultices, tinctures, infusions, decoctions

Cautions: Internal use is restricted in some countries. Do not use on dirty wounds as rapid healing may lead to abscesses

Cloves *Syzygium aromaticum*

Familiar as a culinary spice, cloves are also a useful digestive remedy for nausea and digestive upsets, and are very warming for colds and chills. The oil makes a valuable emergency first aid remedy for toothache and can also relieve insect bites. The Chinese regard cloves as a good kidney tonic helpful for the reproductive organs.

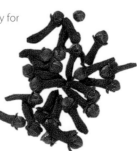

Parts used: Flower buds, essential oil

Actions: Antiseptic, carminative, mild local anaesthetic, warming stimulant, analgesic, antiemetic, antiparasitic

Used in: Massage rubs, lotions, tinctures, infusions

Feverfew *Tanacetum parthenium*

Feverfew is one of the most popular over-the-counter herbs for treating migraine (*see* Headaches and migraine, *page* 134). The plant has been extensively researched since the 1970s and its effectiveness has been demonstrated in a number of clinical trials. It is also a popular over-the-counter remedy for arthritis (*see page* 131) and rheumatism, although many herbs are more effective. As an antispasmodic it can be helpful for period pain and it cools minor fevers.

Parts used: Aerial parts

Actions: Anti-inflammatory, vasodilator, relaxant, digestive stimulant, stimulates menstruation, anthelmintic

Used in: Infusions, tinctures, poultices, fresh leaves, capsules, tablets

Cautions: Do not take if prescribed blood-thinning drugs, such as warfarin. Stop taking if side effects – usually mouth ulceration – occur. Avoid in pregnancy

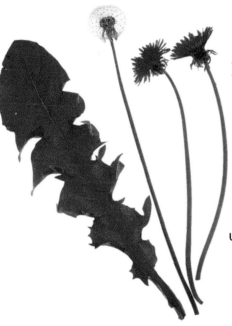

Dandelion *Taraxacum officinale*

Dandelion, a comparative newcomer to Western herbalism, was first mentioned in the 15th century. The plant is strongly diuretic so it is often used for fluid retention (*see page* 111) and urinary problems. The root is also very cleansing for the liver and a mild laxative (*see* Constipation, *page* 120); it is often used in chronic skin problems and arthritis.

Parts used: Leaves, root

Actions: *Leaves:* Diuretic, hepatic and digestive tonic; *Root:* Liver tonic, bile stimulant, diuretic, laxative, antirheumatic

Used in: Infusions, decoctions, tinctures, juices, capsules

Thyme *Thymus vulgaris*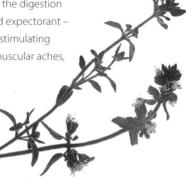

Widely used in cooking, thyme – like many culinary herbs – helps the digestion cope with rich foods. The plant is extremely antiseptic and a good expectorant – ideal to clear phlegm and combat chest infections. The oil is also stimulating and tonifying and can be added to relaxing baths or to rubs for muscular aches, pains and stiffness.

Parts used: Aerial parts, essential oil

Actions: Antiseptic, expectorant, antispasmodic, astringent, antimicrobial, diuretic, antitussive, antibiotic, wound herb, topically rubefacient

Used in: Infusions, tinctures, gargles and mouthwashes, syrups, massage rubs, baths

Caution: Avoid use of essential oil in pregnancy

Lime *Tilia cordata*

Lime flowers are a popular after-dinner tisane in France, where they are taken to encourage relaxation as well as improve the digestion after a meal. The plant is calming for the nerves and can help to reduce high blood pressure (*see page* 90). It is believed to combat the build up of fatty deposits in the blood vessels that can lead to atherosclerosis (*see page* 89).

Parts used: Flowers

Actions: Antispasmodic, diaphoretic, diuretic, sedative, anticoagulant, immune stimulant, digestive remedy

Used in: Infusions, tinctures

Red Clover *Trifolium pratense*

Red clover is mainly used by herbalists as a cleansing remedy for skin problems such as psoriasis (*see page* 143) and eczema. It is a useful expectorant and diuretic helpful for dry coughs and gout, while the fresh flowers can relieve insect bites and stings. The herb was used in the 1930s in cancer therapy and still finds a role in the treatment of breast and skin cancers.

Parts used: Flowers

Actions: Cleansing, antispasmodic, diuretic, possible oestrogenic activity

Used in: Tinctures, compresses, ointments, infusions, syrups, douches, fresh flowers

Fenugreek *Trigonella foenum-graecum*

The potent aroma and taste of fenugreek are familiar from Indian and Middle Eastern cookery and the herb gives a spicy flavour to curries, pickles, and garnishes. The seeds are mainly used in herbal medicine as a warming remedy for stomach and kidney chills, and it can be helpful in late-onset diabetes (*see page* 139) to reduce blood sugar levels. The whole dried plant is used as a tea in modern Egypt as a remedy for spasmodic abdominal pain – due both to digestive upsets and menstruation.

Parts used: Seeds, whole herb

Actions: Anti-inflammatory, digestive tonic, stimulates milk production, locally demulcent, uterine stimulant, hypoglycaemic

Used in: Decoctions, infusions, tinctures, capsules, poultices

Cautions: Avoid in pregnancy as it is a uterine stimulant. Insulin-dependent diabetics should not take the plant without professional advice

Damiana *Turnera diffusa var. aphrodisiaca*

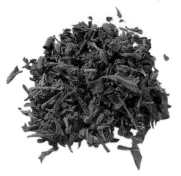

Damiana is a popular aphrodisiac from Central America. It acts as a tonic for the nervous system and antidepressant, but is also stimulating for the digestion and urinary system, useful in convalescence and for general debility. Although largely regarded as a potent male aphrodisiac because of its testosterogenic action, it can be helpful for various menstrual disorders as well.

Parts used: Leaves

Actions: Stimulant, tonic, antidepressant, laxative, diuretic, aphrodisiac testosterogenic

Used in: Infusions, tinctures, capsules, tablets

Slippery elm *Ulmus rubra*

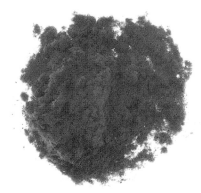

Slippery elm is a highly mucilaginous (sticky) herb mainly used to coat the stomach and provide protection in cases of gastritis (*see page* 120), heartburn (*see page* 121) and ulceration. It is also a valuable nutrient which can be made into a gruel with hot milk and flavoured with honey and spices for convalescents or the seriously debilitated. Used externally it makes an effective drawing ointment for splinters (*see page* 147) and boils and can also soothe wounds and burns.

Part used: Inner bark

Actions: Demulcent, emollient, laxative, nutritive, antitussive

Used in: Capsules, pastes, ointments, poultices, powder (gruel)

Stinging nettle *Urtica dioica*

Nettles 'sting' because the hairs on their stems and leaves contain histamine which is a potent irritant for the skin. However, the plant is a useful tonic, thanks to its ability to rob the soil of relevant nutrients and concentrate minerals and vitamins in its leaves. Nettle makes an ideal spring tonic to cleanse the system and this same action makes it helpful in chronic skin conditions and arthritis. Nettle oil and ointments can be used externally for skin problems and rheumatic pain. The root can be useful for prostate problems (*see* Prostate enlargement, *page* 107).

Parts used: Aerial parts, root

Actions: Astringent, diuretic, tonic, nutritive, haemostatic, circulatory stimulant, stimulates milk production, hypoglycaemic, antiscorbutic

Used in: Infusions, tinctures, ointments, infused oils, capsules, decoctions

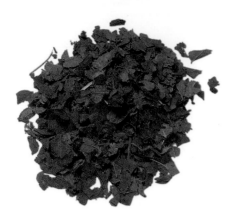

Bilberry *Vaccinium myrtillus*

The fruits are a good source of vitamin C, and are also highly astringent and antibacterial. The fruits are used for diarrhoea, but in large quantities make a palatable remedy for constipation. The fruits are also used externally in salves and ointments for piles, burns and skin complaints. The leaves reduce blood sugar levels and may encourage insulin production.

Parts used: Leaves, fruit

Actions: Astringent, hypoglycaemic, tonic, antiseptic, antiemetic

Used in: Infusions, ointments, tinctures

Caution: Leaves should be avoided by insulin-dependent diabetics unless under professional supervision

Cranberry *Vaccinium macrocarpon*

Cranberry juice has recently been discovered to have an effect on urinary bacteria and is now recommended for urinary infections and cystitis (*see page* 114). The berries are a useful sources of vitamin C.

Parts used: Berries

Actions: Antiscorbutic, urinary antiseptic, diuretic

Used in: Juices, fresh fruits

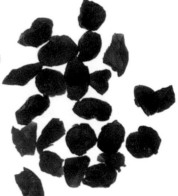

Valerian *Valeriana officinalis*

Valerian is one of the most popular herbal sedatives, used for anxiety and insomnia (*see page* 104). It also reduces high blood pressure (*see page* 90) and is sometimes recommended for a range of heart conditions. It is totally non-addictive and helpful for many stress-related disorders. Extracts are sometimes used in skin creams for eczema.

Parts used: Root and rhizome

Actions: Tranquillizer, antispasmodic, expectorant, diuretic, hypotensive, carminative, mild anodyne

Used in: Decoctions, tinctures, tablets/capsules

Cautions: Excess may cause headache. Do not combine with sleep enhancing drugs

Mullein *Verbascum thapsus*

Mullein is a tall biennial with yellow flowers and leaves that are covered in thick woolly down. It is generally used in soothing cough syrups, while the infused oil, made from the flowers, is helpful for earache (*see page* 90), sores, boils, chilblains and piles. The tall stems were once used to make wicks for candles – hence its common name, candlewort.

Parts used: Flowers, leaves

Actions: Expectorant, demulcent, mild diuretic, sedative, wound herb, astringent, anti-inflammatory

Used in: Infusions, infused oils, tinctures

Vervain *Verbena officinalis*

Vervain was a sacred herb to both Romans and Druids and continued to be associated with magic and fortune-telling until well into the 17th century. Today it is valued as a useful nervine and liver tonic. It is bitter and stimulating for the digestion and makes an ideal tonic in convalescence and when debilitated. Used externally it can ease the pain of neuralgia.

Parts used: Aerial parts

Actions: Relaxant tonic, stimulates milk production, diaphoretic, nervine, sedative, antispasmodic, hepatic restorative, laxative, uterine stimulant, bile stimulant

Used in: Tinctures, infusions, poultices, compresses

Caution: Avoid in pregnancy, although it can be taken in labour to stimulate contractions

Cramp bark *Viburnum opulus*

Cramp bark is a useful relaxant for both the muscles and nerves. It can ease the spasms of cramp and colic and is also helpful for constipation (*see page* 120). It can help with high blood pressure (*see page* 90) by relaxing blood vessels. It can be used externally in creams and lotions to relieve muscle cramps.

Part used: Bark

Actions: Antispasmodic, sedative, astringent, muscle relaxant, nervine

Used in: Decoctions, tinctures, lotions, creams

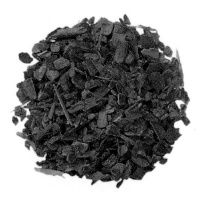

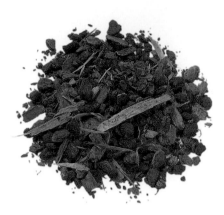

Black haw   *Viburnum prunifolium*   ⚲

Like its relative cramp bark (*see page* 83), black haw is primarily a relaxant useful as an antispasmodic to relieve cramping pains and also to calm the nerves. It seems more specific for the uterus than cramp bark, however, and will rapidly relieve period cramps (*see* Period pain, *page* 120). Herbalists also use the herb for threatened miscarriage and related disorders (*see* Endometriosis, *page* 113).

Parts used: Root bark, stem bark

Actions: Antispasmodic, sedative, astringent, uterine relaxant, diuretic, hypotensive

Used in: Decoctions, powders, tinctures

Heartsease   *Viola tricolor*   ✿ 🌰 🌰

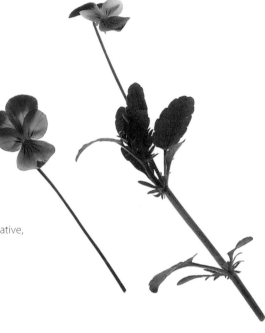

Heartsease, or wild pansy, is a popular garden flower that is good for coughs (*see page* 96), bronchitis and whooping cough, and can soothe skin inflammations and eczema (*see page* 143). It is rich in flavonoids (including rutin) and thus will strengthen capillary walls. Heartsease infusion can be used as a wash to bathe skin sores, nappy rash (*see page* 149), and cradle cap (*see page* 150).

Parts used: Aerial parts

Actions: Expectorant, anti-inflammatory, diuretic, antirheumatic, laxative, stabilizes capillary membranes

Used in: Infusions, tinctures, poultices, creams

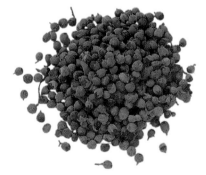

Chaste tree   *Vitex agnus-castus*   ⚲ 🌰

The chaste tree reputedly takes its name from its action as a male anaphrodisiac, used by medieval monks to reduce libido and lascivious thoughts. It was once known as 'monk's pepper' for the same reasons. It acts on the pituitary gland to increase the production of female sex hormones which are involved in ovulation, so it is extremely useful for menstrual irregularities and menopausal problems.

Parts used: Berries

Actions: Pituitary stimulant and hormone regulator, reproductive tonic, increases milk production, female aphrodisiac, male anaphrodisiac

Used in: Tablets/capsules, tinctures

Caution: Excess can create the feeling of ants crawling over the skin

Withania (Winter cherry) (*Ashwagandha*)

Withania somnifera

Known as *ashwagandha* in Hindi, withania or winter cherry is an important Ayurvedic tonic believed to increase vitality and clear the mind. It is mainly used in the West as a tonic for the elderly and to combat debility resulting from overwork and chronic stress. In India it is also used as a tonic in pregnancy.

Part used: Root

Actions: Tonic, sedative, combats stress

Used in: Decoctions, capsules/tablets, powders, tinctures

Cornsilk   *Zea mays*

Cornsilk comprises the long, silky stamens from maize plants which dry to form a crinkled mass resembling red beard clippings. It is a soothing diuretic for an irritated and inflamed bladder and urinary tract disorders, including prostate problems (*see* Prostate enlargement, *page* 107). It can also be helpful for bed-wetting (*see page* 151) in children where this is associated with bladder irritation.

Parts used: Stamens

Actions: Diuretic, soothing for the urinary tract, mild bile stimulant

Used in: Infusions, tinctures, capsules/tablets

Ginger   *Zingiber officinale*

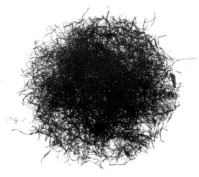

Ginger has been valued as a culinary and medicinal plant since ancient times and is a valuable warming remedy to stimulate the digestion and circulation. In Chinese medicine the dried root is believed to be more helpful for abdominal pain and diarrhoea while the fresh root is more suitable for feverish chills, coughs and vomiting (*see page* 122). As a remedy for nausea (*see page* 122), ginger is ideal for travel sickness (*see page* 152) and has been very successfully tested in clinical trials for severe morning sickness (*see page* 116) in pregnancy. Ginger in capsules or tinctures are ideal, but ginger biscuits or ginger beer can also prove effective, especially with children.

Parts used: Rhizome, essential oil

Actions: Circulatory stimulant, peripheral vasodilator, diaphoretic, expectorant, antiemetic, antispasmodic, carminative, antiseptic.

Topically: Rubefacient

Used in: Decoctions, tinctures, capsules, massage rubs

Caution: Avoid large amounts in cases of gastric ulceration

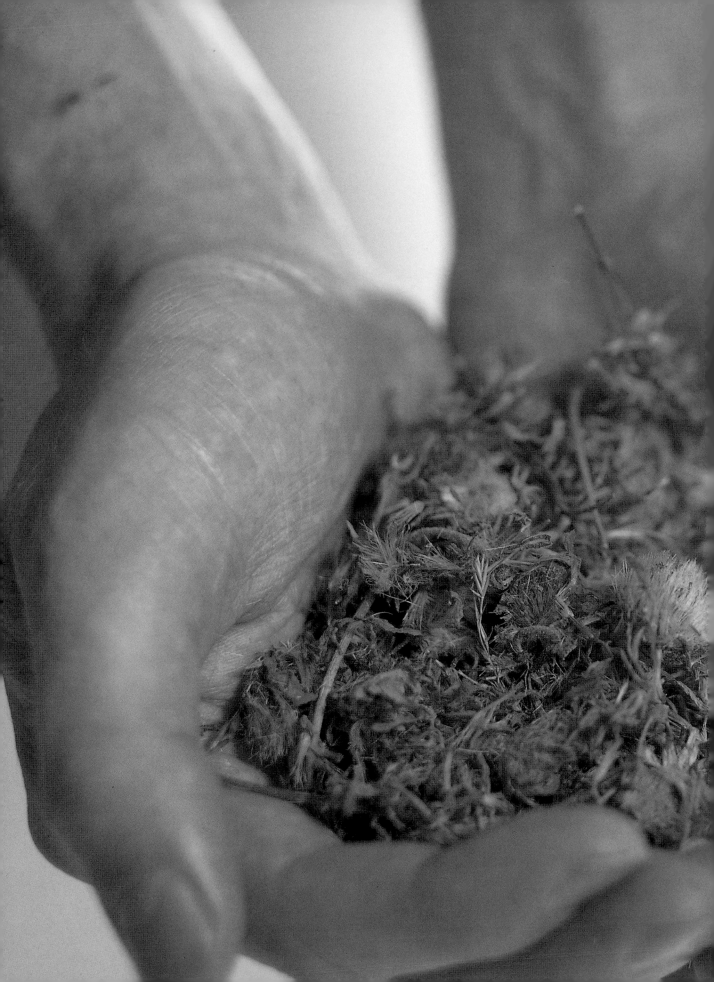

Ailments
solving the problem

Herbs can safely be used at home for a very wide range of ailments – from simply self-limiting problems such as colds or period cramps, to chronic conditions, like arthritis or irritable bowel syndrome. They can also provide a little supportive self-help in more serious conditions and in general will not interfere with orthodox medication. Remember to tell your doctor if you are taking herbal remedies and always check the cautions given in the charts for individual herbs (*see* previous section and safety warnings on pages 5–7 and 116) when taking prescribed drugs.

Heart and circulation

♥ *The high risk of heart disease in the developed world is well known and many people are familiar with the need to relax, take regular exercise, and maintain a low-fat diet. Ancient healing traditions see the heart not as a mechanical pump, but as 'the seat of the soul' and regard modern heart disease as symptomatic of the spiritual vacuum in many people's lives. Herbs like garlic and oats can help reduce blood cholesterol levels; others, like vervain, can provide more holistic support.*

Atherosclerosis

Atherosclerosis is the term used to describe the accumulation of fatty deposits sticking to the walls of the arteries and leads to arteriosclerosis – the hardening of the arteries in old age. Atherosclerosis can also lead to increased risk of blood clots or heart disease if the coronary arteries are affected. It can be linked to excessive smoking and alcohol intake, a fatty diet, pollution, stress (*see page* 101), emotional tension or hereditary weakness. Cholesterol has long been blamed for atherosclerosis, although recent research puts this in doubt. Once established, the fatty deposits tend to be permanent so a healthy diet and relaxed lifestyle are important, especially if there is a family history of heart disease. Likely symptoms include poor circulation (*see page* 91), headaches and giddiness and there could be pain on exertion or breathlessness. Herbs like garlic are useful to thin the blood and lower cholesterol levels, while buckwheat and ginkgo will strengthen blood vessels.

Treatment
- Several herbs can reduce cholesterol levels and may also help to remove the fatty deposits. Make an infusion containing equal amounts of marigold, lime flowers, and hawthorn and drink 1 or 2 cups daily as a preventative.

- Take buckwheat tablets as a source of rutin or make an infusion of buckwheat and drink up to 3 cups daily.

- Take up to 1 gm of garlic daily in capsules or add at least one clove a day, per person, to cooking.

- Ginkgo can also help the circulation and blood vessels – take two 200 mg capsules daily.

- Take 1 tbsp of oatbran each day with your breakfast cereal or sprinkle it on vegetables to help reduce cholesterol levels.

Caution: Self-help remedies and preventatives should be used in conjunction with professional treatment.

Blood pressure problems

The circulation and action of the heart are often compared with simple mechanical systems, such as domestic central heating. Blood is forced around the body in pipes by a pump just like the central heating boiler. Basic laws of physics apply, with pressure proportional to volume: too much fluid and the pressure rises, too little and it falls. When the pipes are narrowed there are similar pressure problems.

Blood pressure is measured with a sphygmomanometer which records the pressure when the heart contracts (systolic) and when it relaxes (diastolic). Although everyone is different and some people have naturally occurring, and quite safe, blood pressure readings that are higher or lower than average, the typical readings for a young, healthy person are 120/80; the average for the over 60s is likely to be 165/85. If the lower reading (diastolic) is above 90 or below 65 then professional investigation may be necessary. Herbs like hawthorn and *Ju Hua* are good for high blood pressure, while low blood pressure often responds more to stimulating tonics.

Seek professional help when

- **There is any sudden or severe chest pain – this needs urgent investigation. Often indigestion is to blame, but it's better to be safe than sorry.**

- **Palpitations continue for more than a couple of minutes, become recurrent, or increase in frequency.**

- **There is dizziness or fainting, especially when standing up or moving from a prone position.**

- **Varicose veins become very red, swollen, and hot as this may indicate thrombosis. This is less apparent with deep veins in the leg, which may only be painful and have a localized hot sensation.**

High blood pressure

The main causes of raised blood pressure include an increase in the thickness of the blood, atherosclerosis (*see page* 89), or kidney disorders, although in 90 per cent of cases there is no obvious cause. Around one in three over-60s are likely to have raised blood pressure. Symptoms can include headaches, nose bleeds (*see page* 98), dizziness and heart pains.

Treatment

- Make an infusion containing equal amounts of hawthorn, *Ju Hua*, yarrow, self-heal, and lime flowers and drink up to 3 cups daily.

- Add a teaspoon of *Ju Hua* flowers to ordinary tea as a pleasant tasting additional supplement.

- Take 20 drops each of cramp bark, hawthorn, and motherwort tincture in water three times a day.

- If stress is a factor, take 10 drops of valerian tincture in water or one 200 mg capsule three times a day.

- Diuretics can be helpful if the problems is linked to fluid retention – drink a dandelion and parsley leaf infusion two or three times daily.

- Take up to 1 gm of garlic in capsules daily.

Caution: Seek professional help for high blood pressure and only use self-help remedies in mild cases. Do not replace long-term blood pressure medication with herbal remedies without first consulting your doctor.

Low blood pressure

Persistent low blood pressure can be associated with blood loss, general debility or shock. Some people have naturally low blood pressure and are none the worse for it: in fact, they generally live longer than average. When low blood pressure becomes a problem the symptoms are likely to include dizziness, headaches, fainting, anxiety (*see page* 101) and panic attacks (*see page* 103). Readings below 110/65 are usually classified as low.

Treatment

- Stimulating herbs can be helpful if debility occurs: take 600 gm of ginseng or damiana daily.

- Make an infusion containing equal amounts of wood betony, peppermint, and rosemary with a pinch of powdered cayenne. Drink 2 or 3 cups daily.

- Eat plenty of oatmeal porridge for breakfast as well as potassium-rich foods like bananas and nuts to improve fluid balance.

- Take kelp and multivitamin supplements.

Supplements

- Garlic, ginkgo, and buckwheat capsules and tablets are widely available from health food shops and pharmacists.

- Vitamin E, an antioxidant, is valuable in all cases of heart and circulatory disorders. Take 400 IU daily. Vitamin E cream can also be used on varicose veins.

- Rutin – which is found in buckwheat – helps to strengthen the blood vessels. Take daily tablets – usually two 200 mg is sufficient.

Palpitations

Awareness of your heart beat can be perfectly normal – especially after vigorous exercise – but sudden palpitations while at rest may be associated with a variety of problems. It could be a sign of anxiety and tension (*see page* 101), be linked to excess caffeine or alcohol, indicate thyroid disorders (*see page* 140) or suggest an underlying heart disorder which may need professional help. Lime flowers and valerian can be especially suitable to bring relief.

Treatment

- If the problem is linked to stress or anxiety then take 10 drops of valerian tincture in a little water; repeat after two hours if necessary. Alternatively, make an infusion of passion flower and drink up to 3 cups daily.

- For general use make an infusion containing equal amounts of motherwort, vervain and lime flowers and drink up to three cups daily.

- Take vitamin E (400 IU) supplements daily.

- Use 2–3 drops of galangal tincture on the tongue to give relief.

- Rose oil can be helpful for panic attacks: use 1 drop to 5 ml/1 tsp of almond oil and massage into the temples. Alternatively, put 2 or 3 drops of rose tincture on the tongue.

- Caffeine and similar compounds are found in tea, coffee and cola drinks; limit total intake to no more than 4 cups a day or drink decaffeinated varieties.

Caution: Seek professional help if the problem is recurrent.

Diet

- Eat plenty of fresh fruits and fibre every day.

- Opinion is divided as to the role of cholesterol in heart and circulatory disorders but it makes sense to avoid too much saturated (animal) fat. Use safflower, sunflower or olive oil for cooking. Some rape seed oils contain a type of fatty acid that can damage heart tissue, so avoid cooking oils which simply say vegetable oil – they often contain a mix of rape seed and other oils.

Poor circulation

While poor circulation can be a sign of more serious heart problems it is often simply an inherited tendency, bringing with it regular bouts of chilblains (*see page* 93) and the likelihood of 'dead' fingers (Raynaud's disease) in cold weather. Poor circulation is also a sign of Buerger's disease which is a smoking-related disorder. A sluggish circulation can also indicate general debility and it is common among the elderly and exhausted. Warming stimulants such as ginger and galangal can be helpful.

Treatment

- Make a decoction using a few slices of fresh ginger or galangal root and two or three cloves. Drink a cup of the hot mixture three times a day.

- Drink a daily cup of buckwheat infusion or take buckwheat tablets to improve the quality of blood vessels.

- Take two 200 mg of ginkgo capsules or tablets daily.

- Keep powdered cayenne in a pepper shaker and use it as a condiment at mealtimes.

- Make an infusion of lime flowers, hawthorn and yarrow and drink three times a day; add a clove to each cup.

Iron-deficiency anaemia

Oxygen is carried to the tissues by haemoglobin in red blood cells and its deficiency leaves the body starved of oxygen, with symptoms of fatigue, breathlessness, pallor, insomnia, dizziness, assorted aches and pains, confusion and reduced resistance to infection. Iron is needed for the body to manufacture haemoglobin so its lack, from poor diet or absorption, can lead to anaemia, in which there are reduced levels of haemoglobin and red blood cells. Loss of blood is also an obvious cause and women who regularly have heavy periods can often suffer from undiagnosed anaemia, leading to general fatigue and recurrent infections. As many as 15 per cent of women regularly suffer from anaemia for this reason. Herbs that are rich in iron such as nettles or parsley are useful, as are Chinese blood tonics, like *Dang Gui*.

Preventatives

- Give up smoking – it has been shown to damage the circulatory system and can lead to arteriosclerosis and Buerger's disease.

- Although a daily glass of red wine is beneficial for the heart and can be a good source of iron, avoid excess alcohol. Current guidelines usually recommend no more than 14 units a week for women and 21 units for men.

- Take regular exercise – it does the heart good to work hard occasionally. People under 50 should try to take at least 20 minutes vigorous exercise three times a week; for older people regular weight bearing exercise (such as gardening or walking home with shopping) is often more beneficial than energetic pursuits such as squash, vigorous running and football.

Treatment

- Take a regular dose of *Dang Gui* to nourish the blood. Use 5 ml/1 tsp of tincture twice a day or else take two 200 mg capsules of the herb daily.

- Bitter herbs can stimulate the digestion and improve iron absorption – take 5 drops of wormwood tincture in a little water before meals.

- Echinacea can help to stimulate red blood cell production – take two 200 mg capsules daily.

- Make an infusion of two parts stinging nettle to one part parsley to make an iron-rich brew. Drink 1 or 2 cups daily.

- Eat plenty of iron rich foods, such as apricots, egg yolk, watercress, liver, kidney and parsley.

- Take Vitamin B_{12} supplements.

Caution: There are many causes of anaemia and professional diagnosis is essential as some – such as leukaemia – can be life-threatening.

Varicose veins

Veins, unlike arteries, have to help force blood back to the heart rather than depend on the impetus of this powerful pump. The muscles surrounding deep veins can help considerably, but the superficial veins in the legs often have little support and over the years they can become distended, lengthened and tortuous. They can ache, feel hot, or the surrounding area can be prone to swelling. A tendency for varicose veins is often hereditary and can also be associated with pregnancy, obesity, standing for long periods, constipation, tight clothing and lack of exercise.

Treatment

- Apply a cream containing melilot and marigold to the affected areas night and morning.

- Take buckwheat tablets or a cup of buckwheat infusion daily.

- Make an infusion containing equal amounts of motherwort, parsley and yarrow and drink a cup two or three times a day.

- Use a lotion containing distilled witch hazel with 10 per cent melilot tincture to ease hot, painful veins.

- Take ginkgo or garlic tablets as a supplement.

- Deep breathing can help encourage the return of blood from the peripheries, while a tendency for varicose veins can often be countered by alternately hosing the legs with a hot and cold shower for 1–2 minutes each morning.

- It can also help to raise the end of the bed to aid venous return (the return of the blood to the lungs for fresh oxygenation via the venous system).

Piles

Piles, or haemorrhoids, are a type of varicose veins (*see left*) which can easily be felt, like bunches of grapes, around the rectum. About 50 per cent of the adult population will suffer from piles at some time in their lives. When piles are severe they can be extremely uncomfortable and make sitting quite painful; they can also bleed and have an associated discharge of mucus. Piles are often linked to constipation (*see page* 120) and over-straining; they are also common in pregnancy (*see page* 116). Herbal laxatives can help, while astringent ointments can be used to help tonify the venous tissue and restore it to normal.

Treatment
- Drink an infusion containing equal amounts of lady's mantle, melilot and buckwheat two or three times a day.

- Use chickweed, silverweed, common plantain or aloe vera ointment on the affected area.

- Use isphaghula as a bulking laxative to avoid constipation – make a maceration of the seeds and drink each morning. Alternatively, mix a teaspoon of seeds with breakfast cereal and add milk, this helps to disguise the rather unpalatable texture of the mix.

- To relieve itching and discomfort make a paste of powdered comfrey in water and apply it to the affected area. Fresh sap from aloe vera leaves can also help or use a poultice of fresh common plantain leaves.

Chilblains

Poor blood flow to the remoter parts of the body, generally in response to cold, is the usual cause of chilblains. In order to maintain a suitably warm temperature for the vital organs and deep tissues of the body, the blood flow to the peripheries is constricted, leading to numbness. As the oxygen supply is limited, the tissues become more alkaline, so that when the temperature does rise and the blood supply returns, the system starts to restore normal balance and the familiar burning and itching sensation of chilblains is the result. Herbal treatment usually combines warming circulatory stimulants – such as ginger or cayenne – with ointments to give symptomatic relief.

Treatment
- Arnica cream is ideal to relieve symptoms: apply a little to chilblains, but only if the skin is unbroken.

- Improve the circulation generally with stimulating herbs. Make a decoction of ginger or galangal and add a small pinch of powdered cayenne – drink 2 or 3 cups a day. Alternatively, drink a cup of rosemary infusion three times a day.

- Rubbing chilblains with a piece of raw onion or lemon juice can also help.

- For chilblains where the skin is broken, use echinacea or chamomile cream.

Ear, nose and throat

Modern medicine tends to blame respiratory problems on infection and pollution, while the dramatic growth in childhood asthma may be linked to both excessive use of antibiotics and car exhaust fumes. In Chinese medicine the lungs are associated with the emotion of grief and this theory argues that chest problems can often follow bereavement, emotional upset or loss. Herbs like elecampane and ginseng are good lung tonics, while others, such as thyme, silverweed or elder, can deal with specific symptoms.

Asthma

In asthma the small bronchial tubes in the lungs tighten, making it difficult for the sufferer to breathe out and leading to the characteristic wheeze. The tubes also fill with a sticky mucus instead of the usual lubricating fluid phlegm. Asthma is often an allergic reaction, so identifying the allergen is important. Dairy products, wheat or beef can be common culprits, while dust and traffic fumes exacerbate the condition. Sulphur dioxide – a common air pollutant – can be to blame, and this same chemical is often used as a preservative for fruits and wine. Emotional stress can also play a part. Herbal remedies usually include relaxing expectorants and antispasmodics (which relieve muscle spasms and cramps) to help ease the symptoms.

Treatment

- A steam inhalation of chamomile can help minimize mild attacks: use 1 tbsp of flowers or 10 drops of chamomile oil to 1 litre/1¾ pints of boiling water.

- Make a chest rub containing 5 drops each of eucalyptus, thyme, and fennel essential oils on 5 ml/1 tsp of almond oil and massage two or three times a day to ease breathing problems.

- Make a decoction of elecampane, liquorice and marshmallow roots and drink a cup two or three times a day.

Caution: Asthma can be life threatening; always seek professional treatment and only use self-help remedies to support orthodox therapy.

Bronchitis

Bronchitis is an inflammation of the bronchial tubes which are the airways bringing air into the lungs. It can be 'acute', due to an infection or 'chronic', which is a serious condition that can lead to lung diseases like emphysema, and is a major cause of early death. While professional medical treatment is usually needed for bronchitis, herbal remedies can also be supportive, with stimulating expectorants to clear the mucus and lung tonics, such as elecampane and ginseng, to strengthen the respiratory system.

Treatment

- Make a decoction containing equal amounts of elecampane and cowslip roots and add 10 ml/2 tsp of horsetail juice to each dose. Drink 2 to 3 cups daily.

- For thick, infected phlegm, take 2 to 3 cups daily of an infusion of thyme, ribwort plantain and marshmallow leaf.

- Use a eucalyptus and thyme oil chest rub – 5 drops of each per 5 ml/1 tsp of almond oil.

- Take up to 600 mg of ginseng daily as a lung tonic.

- It is essential to give up smoking. Alcohol, dairy products, refined carbohydrates, and caffeine should also be strictly limited and avoided altogether if possible.

Caution: Bronchitis often needs professional treatment; only use self-help remedies to support prescribed treatments or in mild attacks.

Seek professional help when

- **There are any problems with breathing or you suffer from chest pains.**

- **Coughs produce blood or blood-streaked phlegm.**

- **Persistent laryngitis or hoarseness occurs as this may indicate a major underlying problem.**

- **Coughs are dry and persistent and unrelated to any recent cold or flu as this can suggest underlying chronic health problems.**

- **Heavy nose bleeds last for several hours – these need to be treated in casualty as soon as possible.**

- **Any condition is accompanied by high temperatures (39°C/102.2°F) which persist for more than a couple of hours.**

- **There is chest pain or tenderness to touch as this may indicate pleurisy or lung damage and needs professional investigation.**

Coughs

Coughing is the body's natural response to any blockage of the airway which may be caused by dust and traffic fumes or mucus resulting from infection. Coughs can be dry and irritating or 'productive', with phlegm varying in shade from white to green. Coloured phlegm generally indicates an infection. Dry coughs can often linger for weeks following a cold and in some cases coughing can become a nervous habit. There is a very wide choice of herbal cough remedies, ranging from the strongly expectorant, which will encourage the production of phlegm, to the cough suppressants, which can ease a persistent dry, tickling cough. Herbal expectorants are sometimes classified as either 'stimulating', which encourage productive coughing, or 'relaxing', which have a more soothing effect and loosen phlegm rather than encouraging its violent removal. Stimulating expectorants include white horehound, cowslip and elecampane. Relaxing expectorants include marshmallow, ribwort plantain, liquorice and hyssop.

Treatment

- For a productive cough use any of the remedies given for bronchitis (see page 95) or make an infusion of mullein, heartsease, white horehound and thyme and drink 3 cups a day. Add 5 ml/1 tsp of honey per cup.

- Use a chest rub containing 5 drops each of peppermint, hyssop and eucalyptus oils in 5 ml/1 tsp of almond oil.

- For irritant dry coughs combine equal amounts of hyssop infusion and liquorice decoction and add the same volume of honey to make a syrup; take 5–10 ml/1–2 tsp up to four times daily.

Caution: Coughing can also be a symptom of more serious illness, so professional medical attention is needed for any cough which persists for more than a few days or where there is no obvious cause.

Catarrh

Catarrh can taken many forms and has many different causes. It is often associated with the common cold (see page 126) and can persist for some time after other symptoms have cleared or it can be a sign of allergic reaction as in hay fever (see right). Catarrh can stay in the upper respiratory tract, causing nasal congestion or the mucus can affect the lower airways and be coughed up as phlegm. Lingering catarrh also makes an ideal breeding ground for bacteria and can lead to inflammation of the sinuses (see Sinusitis, right). While orthodox medicine treats catarrh as a self-contained problem, a more holistic herbal approach regards it as a sign that toxic material elsewhere in the body is not being adequately disposed of – for example the digestive system could be sluggish or the kidneys not working as efficiently as they should. Anti-catarrhal herbs include elder flowers, eyebright, golden seal and ground ivy.

Treatment

- Mix 10 drops each of sandalwood and lavender oil with 5 drops of peppermint oil and use with 1 litre/1¾ pints of boiling water as a steam inhalation or put into a saucer of water for the bedside table at night. An alternative mix can be made from 10 drops of thyme or eucalyptus oil.

- Make an infusion from equal amounts of eyebright, ground ivy, elder flower and silverweed and drink 2 to 3 cups daily.

- Take two 200 mg garlic capsules three times a day or use a clove in cooking.

- Take one 200 mg capsule of powdered golden seal up to three times daily.

- Diet is extremely important and mucus-forming foods, such as refined carbohydrates, dairy products and alcohol, should be avoided. Eating only fruit for a couple of days helps to clear any lingering toxic wastes, while zinc and vitamin C supplements will help to strengthen the immune system and combat infection.

Sinusitis

Severe or persistent catarrh (*see left*) can lead to an inflammation of the sinuses, which are cavities in the bones of the face that help to make the skull lighter. The sinuses are found above the nose, around the eyes,, and across the cheeks, and inflammation can lead to severe localized pain which is made worse by bending forward or blowing the nose. Sinus problems can also be linked to emotional factors: suppressed tears seem to block the upper respiratory tract and a good cry can often be extremely effective.

Treatment

- Combine equal amounts of elder flower, ground ivy, echinacea, silverweed, ginger and peppermint tinctures and take 5 ml/1 tsp three or four times daily in a little warm water.

- Add 5 ml/1 tsp of clove tincture to 1 tbsp of elder flower cream, mix well and massage into sinus areas.

- Take garlic or echinacea supplements to combat infection.

- Use a mixture containing 5 drops each of sandalwood, chamomile, and eucalyptus oils in a steam inhalant two times daily.

- Drink an infusion of elder flower, silverweed and eyebright three times a day: add a pinch of powdered cayenne to each cup.

Diet

- Mucus-forming foods can often encourage catarrh and lead to respiratory tract problems. Limit intake of dairy products, refined carbohydrates and alcohol, and eat plenty of fresh fruit.

- Use garlic regularly in cooking to combat potential infections.

- Pumpkin seeds are a good natural source of zinc, which strengthens the immune system, so add some to salads and use to garnish vegetable dishes.

Hay fever

Although hay fever (allergic rhinitis) is associated with pollen allergies in the summer months, the symptoms can be triggered by a range of problems, including house dust, animal hair and car fumes. Hay fever strictly refers just to symptoms caused by grasses, but many sufferers find that the characteristic sneezing, catarrh and watery eyes start in the spring when flowering currants bloom and continue through to late autumn when the fungal spores arrive. The physical symptoms are largely due to the body's production of histamine (a chemical released during an allergic reaction) as it attempts to rid itself of the allergen, and for this reason orthodox treatments are generally based on antihistamines. The herbal approach involves strengthening the mucous membranes to help reduce the likely allergic response: useful herbs include ribwort plantain, elder flowers, golden seal, ground ivy, chamomile and eyebright.

Treatment

- In early spring take an infusion of equal amounts of elder flower, vervain and white horehound three times a day to help strengthen the upper respiratory tract.

- To relieve symptoms take two 200 mg capsules of eyebright three times a day.

- Bathe the eyes with a weak, well-strained marigold infusion to relieve itching (*also see* Useful eyebaths, *page* 136).

- Use a steam inhalation of chamomile flowers (1 tbsp to 1 litre/1¾ pints of boiling water) if symptoms are severe.

Sore throats

For many people a sore throat can be the first sign of a developing cold or it can suggest pharyngitis, tonsillitis or German measles. The inflammation may be caused by viral or bacterial infection and recurrence can be associated with stress or a reduced resistance to infection. Mild cases often clear in two or three days with or without treatment but the discomfort can be eased by over-the-counter herbal pastilles; gargles are also helpful.

Treatment

- Use a mixture of equal amounts of sage, rosemary and lady's mantle leaves for an infusion, strain well, add 2 drops of cayenne tincture or a small pinch of powdered cayenne and use as a gargle. Repeat every 30–40 minutes if possible.

- Raspberry or agrimony leaf can be substituted for rosemary or lady's mantle and the mix used in the same way.

- Add 5 ml/1 tsp of echinacea tincture to a cup of warm water and use as a gargle.

- Laryngitis and pharyngitis can be helped by steam inhalations containing 5 drops each of sandalwood and lavender oils. Add the same oils to 10 ml/2 tsp of almond oil and massage the external area of the throat.

- Gargle with freshly pressed lemon juice diluted with an equal amount of warm water.

Supplements

- Over-the-counter herbal pastilles and lozenges are useful to ease symptoms. Look for remedies containing hyssop, liquorice, thyme, cowslip, echinacea, fennel, horehound, or cloves. Avoid those with a high proportion of menthol as they can be irritant.

- Honey and lemon is a traditional way to ease sore throats and minor irritant coughs: mix equal amounts of honey and fresh lemon juice and take in 5 ml/1 tsp doses.

- A traditional folk recipe for cough syrup is simply to layer slices of onion or turnip with sugar or honey in a dish and leave overnight. Next morning pour off the liquid and take in 5 ml/1 tsp doses.

- Elder flower cordial makes a useful substitute for infusion – dilute the concentrated mix with hot water and use as an infusion for catarrh (*see page* 96), hay fever (*see page* 98), or sinus problems (*see page* 96).

- Take vitamin C and zinc supplements to strengthen the immune system and combat infection.

Tonsillitis

The tonsils are small packs of lymphatic tissue at the back of the throat which help protect the body from infection. Recurrent tonsillitis can often indicate some underlying food allergy, with the immune system having to work overtime to combat the problem. Herbal gargles can help as a short-term measure.

Treatment
- Add 10 ml/2 tsp each of sage, echinacea and golden seal tinctures to 25 ml/5 tsp of freshly pressed cleavers juice and take a 10 ml/2 tsp dose of the mix three times daily.

- Mix equal amounts of thyme, sage and lady's mantle for an infusion; strain well, and gargle with a cupful when cooled.

- Mix equal amounts of ground ivy, marigold and chamomile for an infusion and drink a cup three or four times a day.

- Add 5 drops each of thyme and hyssop oils and 1 drop of rose oil with 5 ml/1 tsp of almond oil and massage the external neck area. Wrap a warm scarf around the neck. Use the same oils in a steam inhalation.

- Take echinacea or garlic supplements to boost the immune system and combat infection.

Caution: In severe cases the tonsils can become filled with pus, causing an abscess or quinsy which may need surgical treatment. Tonsillitis can be severe and requires professional medical help, especially if it is accompanied by fever.

Nose bleeds

Nose bleeds can often be associated with colds (*see page* 126) and catarrh (*see page* 96), although they can indicate high blood pressure (*see page* 90) so professional help may be needed. Many children suffer regular minor nose bleeds because the delicate blood vessels near the surface of their nose easily become irritated. Many herbs have traditionally been used to stop nose bleeds: the classic example is yarrow, which has the country name of 'nosebleed'.

Treatment:
- Insert a fresh yarrow leaf in the nostril, squeeze the nose gently and lean forward.

- Put a little shepherd's purse or bistort tincture or distilled witch hazel on to a cotton wool swab and insert into the nostril.

Caution: Seek professional help for heavy and/or continual nose bleeds which persist for some hours.

Earache

Ear pain may be linked to catarrh (*see page* 96) and sinusitis (*see page* 97) or there could be a more localized infection and inflammation. Herbal antibiotics and nasal decongestants, such as garlic, plantain and mullein, are ideal for household first aid.

Treatment
- Put the inner heart of a cooled, boiled onion into the ear and secure with a sticking plaster or cotton wool. Alternatively, use a few drops of garlic oil from a capsule on a cotton wool swab.

- Use a few drops of infused mullein oil or fresh common plantain juice on a cotton wool swab and insert it into the ear.

- Make an infusion of marshmallow leaves, elder flower and thyme and drink a cup every three hours.

- Take two 200 mg capsules of echinacea up to four times a day to combat infection.

- Massage the mastoid bone (behind the ear) with a mixture of 10 drops each of lavender and tea tree oil in a 5 ml/1 tsp of almond oil.

Caution: Never put anything into the ear if there is a risk that the drum has perforated. Simple earache will generally resolve within 24 hours, but if it persists seek professional help; do not delay treatment, especially in children.

Glue ear

Secretory otitis media – glue ear – is common in children and can often be associated with milk allergy. It causes fluid to collect in the ear which can lead to deafness, and is characterized by earache (*see above*) and sticky secretions. Orthodox treatment generally involves inserting grommets into the eardrum to relieve pressure.

Treatment
- Make an infusion containing equal amounts of golden rod, ribwort plantain and St John's wort and drink a cup two or three times a day.

- Take one to three 200 mg capsules of golden seal daily (dosage is age dependent, *see page* 152). Alternatively, take 5–20 drops of golden seal tincture in a little water or fruit juice up to three times daily.

- Try a dairy-free diet for at least two weeks.

Toothache

Apart from such obvious damage as a cracked filling or broken tooth, a more likely cause of sudden and severe tooth pain is an abscess or infection. This can often be associated with general feelings of being unwell or perhaps follow a cold. Herbal remedies that stimulate the immune system and counter infections can provide relief and may help disperse abscesses. Persistent toothache – with no obvious dental cause – may be associated with sinus problems (*see page* 97) or catarrh (*see page* 96).

Treatment
- Add a few drops of clove oil to cotton wool and apply to the gum to give emergency pain relief.

- Use echinacea or garlic tablets to boost the immune system and combat infection. Take three 200 mg capsules up to three times a day.

Preventatives

- If you are prone to catarrhal problems, keep a saucer of hot water with 2 or 3 drops of eucalyptus or sandalwood oil in the bedroom, or use an oil diffuser.

- Remember to start hay fever treatments in early spring – before symptoms start.

- Damp, cold weather often encourages respiratory problems and catarrh: drink ginger decoction and elderberry cordial during the winter months and take ginseng for four weeks in late autumn to strengthen the body's natural defences.

Emotions and energy

Mood swings, emotional upsets, and the stressful demands of work and family are all part of normal, everyday life. Usually we cope reasonably well, but everyone – sooner or later – finds it all becomes just too much. Stress usually leads to raised levels of adrenaline – the 'fight or flight' hormone we manufacture to give the body an extra energy boost to cope with emergencies – and this perpetual state of alertness can lead to exhaustion and an inability to relax. Herbs can help to ease the tensions and improve our ability to cope with those stresses.

Stress

Stress is a normal part of our lives and many argue that it is essential to maintain vigour and vitality. Sometimes, however, the stresses can threaten to overwhelm us. If it is proving impossible to cope, then a major reassessment of lifestyle may be necessary. For minor peaks, herbs can provide relief – especially in advance: if a stressful time is looming, such as exams, the school holidays or a heavy work period, then it is worth taking tonic herbs before the event to provide an energy boost rather than depending on short-term stimulants once the stresses mount.

Treatment
- Siberian ginseng is ideal at helping the body to cope more efficiently with stress and improve performance: take up to 600 mg a day for ten to fourteen days before the stresses are due to peak. For long-haul air travel take the same amount for a week before flying to combat jet lag.

- Withania is similarly effective: make a decoction of the root or take up to 600 mg daily in capsules.

Depression

Most of us feel down at some point in our lives, but clinical depression is a serious illness that needs professional help – preferably counselling and psychiatric support rather than potent antidepressant drugs which have side effects and will not necessarily provide a long-term cure. In traditional Galenic medicine (*see page* 12) depression was regarded as 'melancholia' and was the result of too much 'black bile' in the system; it was therefore treated with strong purgatives and digestive remedies. Interestingly, depression is often accompanied by constipation as intense sadness seems to shut down the digestive system as well. The herbal approach generally involves countering any physical exhaustion and debility (*see page* 103) which may be contributing to the problem, stimulating the digestive system if necessary, and strengthening the nervous system. Suitable healing plants include damiana, vervain, ginseng, lemon balm, skullcap, St John's wort and rosemary.

Treatment
- Combine equal amounts of wild oats, lemon balm, St John's wort and vervain tinctures or use the dried herbs for an infusion. Take 5 ml/1 tsp of tincture or 1 cup of infusion three times a day.

- Add 5 drops of basil and sandalwood oils to a daily bath and use the same oils as a massage rub for the throat and chest. Do not use basil oil in pregnancy – substitute lemon balm oil (also known as melissa oil).

- Mix equal amounts of wood betony and basil and use as an infusion three times daily.

- Stimulate the digestion with 2 drops of wormwood tincture in a little water before meals.

Anxiety and tension

For anyone suffering severely from anxiety and tension or who really cannot cope with their lifestyle, self-help herbal remedies are no substitute for professional support. They are ideal for occasional use when the stresses mount and tempers become frayed. Herbal sedatives and tranquillizers also need to be seen as part of a total therapeutic approach: taking herbal relaxants is not going to solve problems caused by overwork and family discord any more than orthodox tranquillizers will. Learning to

Seek professional help when

- **Depression is severe and persistent – sufferers may lack energy or the will to seek help so be attentive of friends and family.**

- **Headaches are severe and persist for more than 48 hours despite medication.**

- **There is any loss of sensation in limbs or restrictions in muscle movements.**

- **There are any visual disturbances, especially double vision.**

relax can be a more effective long-term solution. Herbal nervines, which have a soothing and calming effect on the nerves, fall into a number of categories, including:

- Herbal sedatives and relaxants which can ease tensions and feelings of anxiety.

- Herbs which can act on the emotions in some way.

- Herbal tonics and stimulants which will provide additional short-term energy.

- Energy tonics which will help counter stress by strengthening the system and vital force, increasing a person's ability to cope.

There are a variety of suitable relaxants for anxiety and stress; these include valerian, passion flower, skullcap, vervain, wood betony and chamomile.

Treatment

- Make an infusion containing equal amounts of skullcap, passion flower and wood betony: drink a cup up to four times a day as required.

- Use drops of lemon balm tincture on the tongue or make lemon balm infusion using the fresh herb. Drink a cup up to five times daily.

- Take two 200 mg capsules of valerian twice a day or 20 drops of tincture in a little water for up to three weeks at a stretch.

- Take at least ten minutes each day to practise calm, deep breathing exercises or use a visualization tape to encourage restful meditation if you prefer.

- Relaxing baths can help: add a few drops of basil, hyssop, chamomile or lavender oil to the bath water.

- Take up a relaxing exercise therapy – such as yoga or Tai Ch'i Chuan; don't use aerobics to aid relaxation as it is far too vigorous.

Emotional upsets

Overwrought emotions have many causes, and there are times when we become overwhelmed – by grief, regret, nostalgia, envy – or other powerful feelings. The most widely available herbal remedies for the emotions are the Bach Flower Remedies (*see page* 105) which have been used since the 1930s and are very effective for soothing worries, fears and ill-temper.

Treatment

- Choose the most suitable Flower Remedy and add 5 drops to 10 ml/2 tsp of water; drop the solution on the tongue as needed.

- Make an infusion containing equal amounts of wood betony and chamomile and sip slowly as you calm down.

- Take one 200 mg capsules of reishi up to three times a day.

- Aromatic oils can have a direct impact on the olfactory nerve and centres in the brain involved in emotion. Smelling certain oils can be stimulating and uplifting, while others have a more soothing and relaxing effect. Using oils in diffusers to scent rooms or adding a few drops to bath water can be easy ways to influence the emotions. Try basil, chamomile, lavender, lemon balm, rose or sandalwood.

Diet

- Eat plenty of oatmeal porridge – it is extremely energy giving.

- Ensure adequate intake of green vegetables, nuts and bananas to give B vitamins and blackcurrants, bilberries, cherries and other fruits for vitamin C.

- Eat less refined sugar and carbohydrates.

- Avoid caffeine-containing drinks and limit your alcohol intake.

- Starchy foods – like pasta and grains – are energy giving; also eat plenty of dried fruit and root vegetables to combat tiredness.

- Avoid large meals late at night.

Exhaustion and fatigue

General tiredness is one of today's most common complaints. Our society is often described as 'cash rich, time poor' and we all try to do too much in too little time. The result is often a general lack of energy that falls short of clinical exhaustion but can interfere with enjoyment and performance. Herbal stimulants are, of course, familiar to all: coffee, tea, cola drinks and chocolate are all rich in caffeine and related alkaloids, and act as a short-term restorative. Herbs can also provide a longer-term energy boost

Treatment

- Take up to 600 mg daily of Siberian ginseng, *Dang Gui,* ginseng, or withania capsules for up to four weeks. In general *Dang Gui* and Siberian ginseng tend to be more suitable for women.

- Make an infusion of rosemary and gotu kola tea and drink up to 3 cups daily.

- Eat a bowl of oatmeal porridge for breakfast each day – it is very energy giving.

- Add 5 drops of rosemary, thyme or sandalwood oils to bath water.

Debility

Weakness and lack of vitality may follow an illness or be associated with overwork and undernourishment. Low blood pressure (*see page* 90) is commonplace. Debility can also be associated with a number of underlying chronic conditions, including anaemia (*see page* 92), so seek professional help if there seems to be no obvious reason for the weakness.

Treatment

- Make an infusion containing equal amounts of agrimony, wild oat straw and chamomile flowers – drink a cup three times daily.

- Take *Dang Gui* – 5 ml/1 tsp of tincture three times a day or up to 600 mg of capsules daily.

- Make a decoction containing equal amounts of ginseng root, liquorice root and withania or use supplements of these herbs in capsule form (up to 600 mg daily of any of them).

- Ensure that your diet contains an adequate intake of vital minerals and vitamins; alfalfa sprouts, kelp and multivitamin tablets are useful supplements.

Panic attacks

These can often be related to palpitations (*see page* 91) or may be associated with anxiety and tension (*see page* 101). As well as breathing problems and general feelings of panic there may be pallor and sweating.

Treatment

- Take 1 drop of rose oil on a sugar lump, or add 2 drops of rose oil to a diffuser to scent the room

- Make an infusion of wood betony and skullcap tea and sip it slowly until you feel calmer.

Shock

Shocks from sudden fears or physical trauma are generally typified by a cold sweat, rapid pulse, breathlessness, giddiness and shivering. Keeping warm, ideally in bed, is best, while the traditional remedy of a hot cup of tea does much to restore fluid balance.

Treatment

- Drink a cup of an infusion containing equal amounts of lime flowers and skullcap.

- Use a few drops of Bach Flower Rescue Remedy (*see page* 105) directly on the tongue.

- Take a cup of slippery elm gruel (1 tsp powdered slippery elm and hot milk) as a restorative.

- Use a few drops of rosemary oil in an oil diffuser to scent the room.

Caution: For severe shock following an accident seek emergency medical attention. Give no food or drink to people in severe shock.

Insomnia

There are no hard and fast rules as to how much sleep we need, but sleeplessness becomes a problem when sufferers feel tired and unable to concentrate during the day or when it becomes a worry in itself, with seemingly endless hours spent tossing and turning in bed at night. Usually the body will catch up eventually and a few bad nights are often followed by a period of restful and restorative sleep. There are many causes for insomnia – heavy meals late at night that disturb the digestion, painful joints and muscles or irritating coughs. Often insomnia is associated with tension and worries and a failure to relax before bedtime.

Treatment
- Make an infusion of cowslip flowers, Californian poppy and passion flower; drink a cup 30 minutes before bed. Alternate with a mix of lemon balm, lavender and lime flowers.

- Fill a small cushion with freshly dried hops and put under the pillow at night.

- Mix 10 ml/2 tsp each of hops, lavender and cowslip flower tincture and take 10 drops in a little water at night. Leave a second dose on the bedside table for use during the night.

- Take ready-made tablets or capsules containing valerian, passion flower, hops, lavender, lime flowers or chamomile – these are available in various combinations.

- Eat oatmeal porridge daily to combat nervous exhaustion that can follow sleeplessness.

Preventatives and lifestyle

- Find time for yourself – at least 30 minutes every day spent doing what you want to do, not what family and work demands dictate.

- Take a relaxing bath with a few drops of lavender or basil oil at night time to help relax. A morning bath containing a few drops of rosemary oil will energize and invigorate.

- Avoid aggressive exercise regimes, like aerobics, and opt for gentler relaxation therapies, country walks or gardening.

Chronic fatigue syndrome

Myalgic encephalomyelitis (ME) has been dismissed by many as 'yuppy flu' with scant regard to sufferers' problems. Sometimes the symptoms may be influenced by psychological factors – also true for many illnesses. The problem often starts after a viral illness (hence another name – post-viral fatigue) and may involve viral material entering the muscles and causing general weakness and pains. In other cases there may be depression (*see page* 103), weakened immunity, headaches, dizziness or difficulty breathing and a tendency to sleep all of the time. Symptoms can continue for months or even years, and then suddenly vanish.

Treatment
- Strengthen the immune system with echinacea, reishi or *Huang Qi* supplements – take two 200 mg capsules up to four times a day.

- Use cleansing herbs to clear toxins from tissues: take 10 ml/2 tsp of cleavers juice with 1–2 drops of wormwood three times daily.

- Make an infusion containing equal amounts of ginkgo, gotu kola and St John's wort and drink a cup three times daily.

- Take ginseng or withania in capsule form – up to 600 mg daily.

- Take evening primrose oil (500 mg), vitamin C (500 mg) and zinc and magnesium as supplements daily.

Neuralgia

Neuralgia (nerve pain) can occur anywhere in the body. It is most common as an inflammation of the trigeminal nerve which runs along the side of the face and scalp. The pain is often exacerbated by cold and draughts and in very severe cases surgical treatment is recommended to cut the nerve.

Treatment
- Make an infusion of equal amounts of vervain and St John's wort, add a pinch of powdered ginger or cayenne or a clove and drink up to 5 cups daily.

- Gently apply a warm compress soaked in a lavender, melilot, vervain or St John's wort infusion.

- Use a fresh slice of lemon as a poultice. Alternatively, use 5 drops of lemon oil in warmed almond oil.

The Bach Flower Remedies

Dr Edward Bach identified 38 healing flower extracts in the 1930s. These are still widely used today, although more exotic essences – such as gem extracts and Australian bush plant derivatives – have also joined the repertoire. The Bach Flower Remedies are plant extracts preserved with brandy and are diluted further before being taken in drop doses as required.

Remedy	Dr Bach's suggested use
Agrimony	For those who suffer mental torture behind a 'brave face'
Aspen	For vague fears of an unknown origin
Beech	For critical intolerance of others
Centaury	For the weak-willed
Cerato	For those who doubt their own judgment and seek advice of others
Cherry Plum	For fears of mental collapse
Chestnut Bud	For a refusal to learn from past mistakes
Chicory	For possessiveness and selfishness
Clematis	For the inattentive and dreamy escapist
Crab Apple	A cleansing remedy for those who feel unclean or ashamed
Elm	For those temporarily overcome by feelings of inadequacy
Gentian	For the despondent and easily discouraged
Gorse	For hopelessness and despair
Heather	For the self-centred, obsessed with their own troubles
Holly	For those who are jealous, angry, or feel hatred for others
Honeysuckle	For home sickness and nostalgia
Hornbeam	For 'Monday morning feelings' and procrastination
Impatiens	For the impatient
Larch	For those who lack confidence
Mimulus	For fear of known things
Mustard	For deep gloom and severe depression

Remedy	Dr Bach's suggested use
Oak	For those who struggle on against adversity
Olive	For complete exhaustion
Pine	For guilt feelings and self-blame
Red Chestnut	For excessive fear for others, especially loved ones
Rock Rose	For extreme terror
Rock Water	For the self-repressed who overwork and deny themselves any relaxation
Scleranthus	For uncertainty and indecision
Star of Bethlehem	For shock
Sweet Chestnut	For extreme anguish; the limit of endurance
Vervain	For tenseness, over-enthusiasm, and over-effort
Vine	For the dominating and inflexible
Walnut	Provides protection at times of change such as the menopause or during other major life-stage transitions
Water Violet	For the proud and reserved
White Chestnut	For mental anguish and persistent nagging worries
Wild Oat	For uncertainty about which path to take; an aid to decision taking
Wild Rose	For the apathetic who lack ambition
Willow	For the resentful and bitter who are fond of saying 'not fair'

Male reproductive and urinary tract disorders

♂ *Men are often reluctant to seek help for any health problems, and when it comes to disorders involving the reproductive system they can be doubly reluctant. Prostate cancer often goes undiagnosed, because of this it is important to investigate any symptoms such as a change in patterns of urination. The Chinese argue that the reproductive energy, or Qi, resides in the kidneys and suitable warming herbal tonics can be helpful in many conditions.*

Impotence

Stress, overwork, alcohol and excess caffeine can all contribute to low libido. In chronic conditions professional help is often needed, but more often than not a more relaxed approach to lovemaking will be enough. For many men, doubts about their performance are enough to prevent satisfactory erection and orgasm. In other cases the explanation may be physical – painful piles (*see page* 107) are a common cause. For centuries many herbs have been regarded as aphrodisiacs and although some of these traditional remedies are of doubtful efficacy a few do have a demonstrable effect on the body's hormones. Others are efficient energy tonics to boost inner vital strengths.

Treatment

- Take up to 600 mg of ginseng daily; traditionally it should only be taken in four week periods at most, except in the elderly who can take it all-year round.

- Withania can also be effective – take up to 600 mg in capsules daily.

- Damiana is one of the most popular male aphrodisiacs: take a cup of an infusion three times a day; add one clove per cup to stimulate the system.

- Saw palmetto is effective at increasing sexual stamina and potency: combine tinctures of saw palmetto, damiana and withania and take 5 ml/1 tsp in water twice a day.

- Use 1 drop of rose oil and 5 drops of sandalwood in 5 ml/ 1 tsp of almond oil as body massage for both partners prior to lovemaking. Heat the same oils in a diffuser in the bedroom.

Infertility

Male infertility is generally associated with a low sperm count, and recent studies suggest that too much junk food and contaminants in the form of pesticides can contribute to the problem. Sperm is also damaged by high temperatures – wearing loose trousers rather than tight jeans can help to keep the testes cool. Herbs can help to stimulate sperm production: in traditional Chinese medicine the 'reproductive *Qi*' – the energy needed – is stored in the kidneys, so warming kidney tonics like clove and *He Shou Wu* can be helpful.

Treatment

- Make a decoction containing *He Shou Wu* root and cloves and add half as much liquorice root. Drink a cup three times a day. Use tinctures as an alternative and take 5 ml/1 tsp at each dose. These herbs can also be used in a tonic wine (*see page* 34). Put the roots into a large crock and cover with red wine. Leave for two weeks and then take 1 sherry glass daily.

- Take up to 600 mg of withania in capsules daily.

- If stress (*see page* 101) is contributing to the problem, drink 1 or 2 cups of skullcap, vervain or chamomile infusion each day.

- Eat organically grown produce wherever possible and cut down on alcohol, caffeine and smoking.

Seek professional help when

- **There is difficulty in urination or blood in the urine.**

- **Urination increases in frequency, especially at night.**

- **Urinary infections do not improve within three days or are accompanied by fever.**

- **There is low back pain: this suggests pain in the kidney, especially if following a urinary infection.**

- **There is severe pain from 'loin to groin', suggesting kidney stones or urinary gravel.**

Prostate enlargement

The prostate gland is one of the male sex organs and opens into the urethra, below the bladder. It produces an alkaline fluid which is contained in semen. With age the gland often becomes enlarged, causing problems with passing water: the flow is reduced and residual urine often remains in the bladder, leading to infection. Urine can also travel back from the bladder to the kidneys because of pressure differences, and can cause damage and reduced kidney function. Benign prostate enlargement is thought to be caused by an accumulation of the male sex hormone testosterone in the prostate, where it is converted to a potent chemical called dihydrotestosterone (DHT) which causes the enlargement. Orthodox treatment is usually to remove part of the prostate gland, but the remnants will still retain the tendency to grow so the treatment may need to be repeated. Herbal remedies concentrate on restoring the body's chemical balance by reducing production of DHT and combating any resulting infections.

Treatment
- Saw palmetto berries are a proven treatment for benign prostate enlargement and have been shown to reduce DHT levels. Combine two parts each of saw palmetto and Siberian ginseng tinctures with one part white deadnettle and take 5 ml/1 tsp in water three times a day.

- Take two 200 mg of echinacea capsules up to three times a day to combat any infection caused by lingering urine.

- Drink a cup of an infusion containing equal amounts of corn silk, white deadnettle, and buchu as a healing diuretic. Add 5 ml/1 tsp of horsetail juice to each cup.

- Take 500 mg of evening primrose oil daily.

- Stinging nettle tea can also be beneficial – drink a cup of an infusion (aerial parts) or decoction (root) twice a day.

Caution: There is always the possibility of prostate cancer in any case of prostate enlargement so professional diagnosis is important.

Prostatitis

Inflammation of the prostate gland may be due to bacterial infection. Symptoms are very similar to urethritis (*see below*), with pain and discomfort on passing urine and possible high temperature or fever.

Treatment
- Make an infusion containing equal amounts of horsetail, white deadnettle, and golden rod and drink a cup three times daily.

- Take two 200 mg of garlic in capsules three times a day.

Cystitis and Urethritis

Cystitis simply means inflammation of the bladder while urethritis is an inflammation of the urethra – the tube through which urine is excreted. The first is more common in women, since their urethras are much shorter than men's: around 3.5 cm/1⅜ in compared with about 20 cm/8 in for men. Cystitis affects around half of all women at some point during their lives. Specific urethritis is associated with sexually transmitted disease, and needs treatment at special clinics, while nonspecific urethritis (NSU) is a common problem for men. Symptoms include pain or a burning sensation when passing urine, difficulty urinating, and a dull ache in the lower abdomen. Like all opportunist infections, the bacteria causing the problem are more likely to attack when sufferers are tired, overworked, or under additional emotional stress. To make the acidic urine more alkaline, limit your meat intake, avoid acidic foods like rhubarb, oranges, and pickles and opt for more vegetarian dishes.

Treatment
- Make an infusion containing equal amounts of buchu, yarrow, ground ivy, and golden rod and drink a cup up to four times daily. In severe cases inflammation may lead to blood in the urine – add shepherd's purse to the mixture if this occurs.

- Combine equal amounts of horsetail, marshmallow root and white deadnettle tinctures; take 5 ml/1 tsp three times a day.

- Parsley and dandelion are effective diuretics to help flush the system: drink 3–4 cups of an infusion of either each day. Add a pinch of baking soda to each cup to help reduce the acidity of the urine.

- Take two 200 mg of echinacea capsules three times a day to combat infection.

Caution: Seek professional help if symptoms are severe or persistent. If urethritis is sexually transmitted it must by law (in the United Kingdom) be referred to a doctor.

Urinary gravel

Urinary gravel is formed from deposits of either uric acid or calcium salts which crystallize from solution when the urine is highly concentrated. They then collect in the urinary tract and cause discomfort. Urine tends to be cloudy and passing water feels uncomfortable or gritty. There may also be blood in the urine and severe pain from the perineum down to the thighs. Calcium stones can be more common in hard water areas: either use boiled water or low-calcium mineral water if you have a tendency to urinary gravel.

Treatment
- Combine celery, marshmallow leaves and corn silk in an infusion to encourage urination and to help clear uric acid. Drink a cup up to four times daily. If there is blood in the urine, add shepherd's purse to the mix.

- Take 10 ml/2 tsp of fresh cleavers juice with 5 drops of valerian tincture three times a day.

- Drink cups of a parsley infusion at regular intervals.

- Changing the acidity of the urine can help: eat less meat and more vegetarian meals. Avoid foods with a high oxalic acid content – especially rhubarb, chocolate and spinach. Avoid dairy products which, of course, contain calcium.

Caution: Seek professional help in severe cases. Kidney stones passing from the kidney to the bladder are excruciating – typically it is described as travelling from 'loin to groin' – and may lead to fainting or collapse. Seek professional help in all cases.

Supplements and diet

- Ensure adequate intake of B vitamins, vitamin E, and zinc for all male reproductive disorders: eating pumpkin seeds regularly is a good way to increase zinc intake.

- Drink plenty of fluids for all urinary problems; drink at least 1¾ litres/3½ pints a day – most of it should be water (low calcium mineral water if in a hard water area).

- Include parsley, celery, and dandelion leaves in your diet.

- Eat wholemeal bread and rice-based cereals to ensure adequate fibre intake.

- Drink diluted cranberry juice rather than fruit juices. Sweeten with a little honey if preferred.

- Reduce meat intake to increase alkalinity of the urine: try to have at least three meatless days each week.

- Limit intake of salt and avoid preserved and smoked foods.

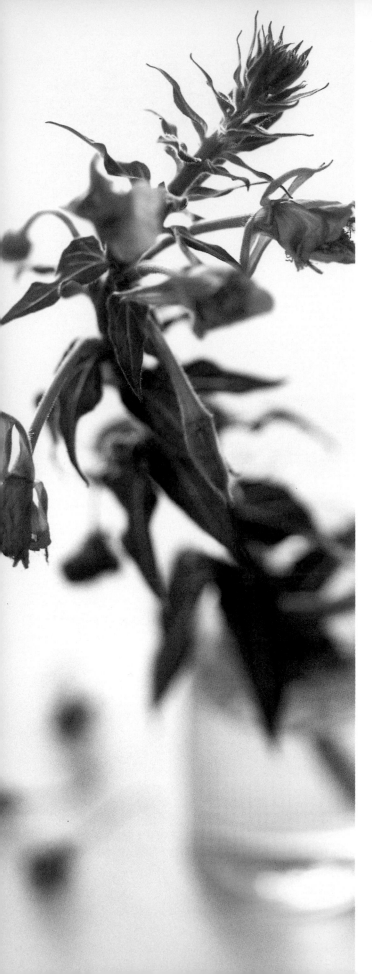

Female reproductive problems and pregnancy

♀ *Herbs have been a vital standby for a vast array of female health problems for centuries: their very names tell us so. Motherwort, lady's mantle, squaw vine* (Mitchella repens), *and mother's hearts* (Capsella bursa-pastoris) *are all names of plants which can be used for gynaecological problems or during pregnancy and childbirth. Chinese medicine associated menstruation with liver function and blood, so herbs like* Dang Gui *– an important female tonic – are also good for the liver.*

Period problems

Premenstrual syndrome

Premenstrual syndrome (PMS) responds well to herbal remedies. Symptoms can include abdominal bloating (*see below*), emotional disturbances, and breast tenderness (*see page* 113). The problem tends to be associated, in orthodox terms, with a too rapid fall in progesterone levels in relation to oestrogen. Conventional treatments concentrate on hormone levels and chaste tree and helonias make ideal herbal remedies. Herbalists, however, tend to regard PMS as rather more multi-dimensional than simply a case of hormones out of balance. Chinese medicine, for example, considers menstruation as involved with liver function and PMS remedies focus on energizing and tonifying this organ using herbs like *Dang Gui*. Evening primrose oil has almost become a herb of choice for many PMS sufferers in recent years. The gamma-linolenic acid (GLA) it contains is believed to help with the production of the prostaglandin E_1 and it can be particularly helpful for relieving fluid retention and breast tenderness. Borage (starflower) oil acts in a similar way.

Treatment

- Make a combined infusion/decoction containing 20 gm of *Dang Gui* and black cohosh root, use 5 gm of liquorice root and fresh ginger root in the decoction and 10 gm each of vervain and yarrow for the infusion. Drink a cup three times daily.

- Take 500 mg daily of evening primrose or borage oil capsules; increase to 1 gm in the ten days before a period is due.

- Take 10 drops of chaste tree tincture in water each morning; increase to 20 drops in the ten days before the period is due.

- Take 20 drops of helonias tincture in water three times a day.

- Cut down on caffeine intake and try to avoid excess stress in the ten days prior to a period.

Fluid retention

Fluid retention is commonly associated with premenstrual syndrome (PMS) (*see above*) and abdominal bloating and is generally best treated by occasional use of diuretic teas. In more severe cases ankles, fingers and hands may swell and there may be palpitations (*see page* 91) and headaches (*see page* 135).

Treatment

- Drink an infusion of parsley, dandelion leaf and buchu or yarrow tea. Add half as much motherwort to the mix if palpitations are also a problem.

- Many over-the-counter tablets are sold for water retention: look for those containing dandelion, horsetail or yarrow and avoid long-term use of those containing juniper, which may damage the kidneys.

- Soak a compress in a lavender infusion and use to relieve aching ankles that have swollen in hot weather.

Caution: Fluid retention can also suggest diabetes (*see page* 139) or heart disorders (*see* High blood pressure, *page* 90) so seek professional help for a sudden onset or a changed pattern of symptoms. Do not take proprietary herbal remedies for fluid retention if you are suffering from raised blood pressure without professional advice.

Seek professional help when

- **There is any severe abdominal or pelvic pain.**

- **There is any significant change in the pattern of menstruation, such as irregularity, increased flow, or bleeding between periods.**

- **You are pregnant or believe you may be – do not take any remedy until you have discussed the matter fully with your doctor.**

- **There are changes in breast or nipple shape, lumps, or swelling in the armpit.**

- **In pregnancy you suffer from prolonged bouts of nausea and frequent vomiting, fluid retention lasting more than three days, breast pain and soreness, and frequent urination or discomfort lasting for more than three days. Ensure regular blood pressure checks throughout.**

Heavy periods

Excessive menstrual bleeding is a common problem, although it is a difficult one to assess as some women always have a heavy flow and consider it quite normal. It is important to seek professional help if there is any change in the established pattern of menstruation as it could be related to some underlying cause – such as fibroids or endometriosis (see page 114). Sadly, the orthodox reaction to women who complain of excessive flow (with no apparent cause) is to recommend surgery – often a hysterectomy. The latter can be a mistake: in Ayurvedic theory the womb is closely associated with the energy centres or chakras of the body and its removal often leads to unexpected emotional upsets. Shepherd's purse and marigold are among the many useful herbs which can help avoid such traumas.

Treatment

- Make an infusion containing equal amounts of shepherd's purse, lady's mantle, marigold and raspberry leaf and drink 2 cups daily; increase to 4 cups during menstruation.

- Heavy periods are a common contributory cause of anaemia: take two 200 mg capsules of Dang Gui daily to combat the risk. Eat plenty of iron-rich foods (see Iron-deficiency anaemia, page 92).

- Take 10 drops of chaste tree tincture in water each morning to help normalize hormonal activity.

- Make an infusion containing equal amounts of white deadnettle and stinging nettles and drink 1 or 2 cups a day instead of tea or coffee. Flavour with honey or lemon juice if preferred.

Irregular/scanty periods

Irregular periods can be associated with poor nutrition and low body weight – a common problem for both anorexics and ballet dancers. Pregnancy is another obvious cause for absent periods, so do take a pregnancy test before starting on stimulating medication. Other causes include trauma, fibroids (see right) and anaemia (see page 92). Many herbs can stimulate menstruation, and were used in the past to cause miscarriage. This is a dangerous practice as such attempts are more likely to lead to a damaged foetus than to an abortion. Absent periods are believed to increase the risk of premature osteoporosis.

Treatment

- Take 10 drops of chaste tree tincture in water each morning.

- Combine equal amounts of helonias, black cohosh and motherwort tinctures. Take 5 ml/1 tsp three times a day.

- Drink an infusion containing equal amounts of motherwort, yarrow and rosemary up to three times a day.

- If thyroid imbalance (see page 140) is a contributory factor take kelp tablets as a supplement.

- Take supplements of B vitamins and vitamin E as well as additional zinc.

Period pain

A number of herbs are used for period pain and their choice will depend on the nature of the discomfort. Herbalists tend to divide period pain into:

- Congestive pain which builds up shortly before the period starts. It is associated with blood stagnation and blood congestion and can involve bloating and fluid retention (see page 111). It eases once the period has begun.

- Spasmodic pain due to uterine cramps which begins once flow starts and can be linked to a prostaglandin imbalance and emotional tension.

Motherwort and helonias will ease the stagnation sort of pain while black haw and black cohosh are better for cramping pain.

Treatment

- Take 20 ml/4 tsp of black haw tincture in water for cramping pain. Usually one dose is sufficient but it may be repeated after four hours if necessary.

- Make an infusion combining equal amounts of St John's wort, silverweed, motherwort and raspberry leaf. Drink a cup three times a day. A cup of passion flower infusion may also be helpful.

- Take 40 drops of helonias tincture in water three times a day for stagnation pain.

- Mix 5 drops each of rosemary and basil oils in 5 ml/1 tsp of almond oil and massage the abdomen between the navel and the pubic area.

Breast discomfort and benign lumps

Painful, swollen breasts are commonplace in the days before a period; indeed many women even have to wear a larger bra at those times because the swelling is so significant. Fibrocystic breast disease (FBD) involves the formation of numerous small benign cysts, often with no other symptoms. Both problems are very common. Herbal treatments for PMS can often help.

Treatment

- Diuretics can help to remove the excess fluids contributing to swollen breasts and breast lumps. Make an infusion containing equal amounts of cleavers, parsley and horsetail and drink 1 cup morning and evening.

- Take 1 gm of evening primrose oil in capsules daily.

- Apply a compress soaked in horsetail and cleavers infusion to sore breasts if necessary.

- Take beta-carotene supplements or drink a glass of carrot juice daily.

Supplements and diet

- Evening primrose and borage (starflower) oil are good sources of gamma-linolenic acid (GLA); take up to 1 gm daily for menstrual and menopausal problems; combinations including fish oils can be helpful at the menopause.

- Ensure adequate intake of B vitamins and zinc; use supplements if your diet is likely to be deficient. Vitamin B$_6$ has been recommended for PMS but there are now doubts about its safety – do not exceed dosages given on packs.

- Avoid all caffeine drinks.

- Limit sugar intake and keep alcohol intake to a minimum.

Caution: Although any link between FBD and breast cancer is unproven, it is best to have any breast lump investigated. FBD sufferers who are used to their lumpy breasts should be alert for any change in the character of lumps.

Endometriosis

This is where tissue normally found lining the womb (the endometrium) leaks into the pelvic cavity and can lead to obstructions and tissue change. Adhesions may affect the uterus and the bowel; the result is heavy and painful periods, and sometimes diarrhoea or constipation. The condition may disappear during pregnancy or at the menopause. It can affect fertility and the chances of conception; orthodox treatment tends towards surgery but herbs can provide an alternative for relieving the symptoms.

Treatment

- Combine equal amounts of wild yam, vervain, black haw, marigold, dandelion root and hawthorn berry tinctures, and take 5 ml/1 tsp three times a day.

- Drink a chamomile, marigold and St John's wort infusion with a pinch of powdered ginger to relieve discomfort.

- Take 10 drops of helonias tincture in water three times daily.

Caution: Endometriosis often requires professional treatment; do not depend on self-help.

Fibroids

Fibroids and non-malignant growths in the uterus usually give no pain, but they are associated with heavy menstrual bleeding. They are a common cause of infertility and in severe cases may lead to a hysterectomy. They are related to oestrogen levels and have been associated with use of the contraceptive pill. After the menopause, when oestrogen levels fall, fibroids tend to shrink naturally. Herbal treatment can be successful in helping to shrink the growths, but it often takes time so do not be rushed into the surgical option too quickly.

Treatment

- Make an infusion containing equal amounts of cornsilk, shepherd's purse and marigold petals; drink a cup three times a day.

- Combine tinctures of golden seal, yarrow, galangal and blue cohosh; take 5 ml/1 tsp three times a day.

- Add 20 drops of golden seal tincture to 1 litre/1¾ pints of boiled water and use as a vaginal douche.

Caution: Seek professional help for any significant increase in the pattern of menstrual flow.

Thrush and vaginal itching

Vaginal thrush is generally caused by *Candida albicans* – a yeast infection responsible for candidiasis (*see page* 123). Like candidiasis, thrush usually starts when the body is out of balance and resistance is low. Typical symptoms are irritation, soreness, characteristic white patches on the membrane lining and a white, cheesy discharge. High blood sugar levels will also encourage yeast proliferation, so the problem can be especially commonplace with diabetics (*see page* 139), while non-diabetics should reduce sugar intake to a minimum. Use of antibiotics also wipes out many of the bacteria which keep the more opportunist yeasts like *Candida albicans* under control, so thrush can often follow another infection and antibiotic treatment.

Treatment

- Put a few drops of tea tree oil diluted in 5 ml/1 tsp of water onto a tampon and insert into the vagina; leave for no longer than 4 hours and repeat twice a day.

- Ease vaginal itching with marigold and lady's mantle cream with 1 drop of rose oil added per dose. Fresh aloe vera sap is also effective.

- Yeasts thrive in warm, damp conditions and thus women prone to repeated vaginal thrush infections should wear cotton pants with cotton gussets and stockings instead of tights to ensure that the perineum remains cool and dry.

- Taking a *Lactobacillus acidophilus* supplement or eating live yoghurt when on a course of antibiotics can help.

- Eat plenty of garlic.

Infertility

For many women the struggle to conceive becomes an all-consuming preoccupation. Modern fertilization techniques can be very successful, but they are often invasive and unpleasant and require dedication by both partners. Herbs can help to improve general health and readiness for conception and be generally supportive, but they are not a magic formula with guaranteed success. Any woman trying to conceive should avoid taking unnecessary medication and ensure that her diet contains sufficient minerals, vitamins and other nutrients.

Treatment

- Make an infusion containing equal amounts of red clover flowers, stinging nettles, peppermint and marigold petals. Drink a cup three times a day.

- Take 5 drops of helonias tincture daily in warm water.

- Take up to 600 mg of *Dang Gui* capsules daily to stimulate the system on the ten days following each period, but do not take them if there is a chance you may be pregnant.

- Thrush and infections can affect fertility, so avoid orthodox antibiotics and take a 200 mg echinacea capsule or 5 ml/1 tsp of echinacea tincture in water instead.

Loss of libido

Just as stress, overwork, alcohol, and excess caffeine can contribute to male impotence, so too with women. The rhythm of the menstrual cycle also plays its part, with libido often tending to rise mid-cycle, just prior to ovulation, and again before menstruation when pressure from the thick endometrium stimulates sexual activity. At other times it can be quite natural to feel less like sexual intercourse and partners should respect this. Where low libido does become a problem, then there are many stimulating herbs to help.

Treatment

- Take 10–20 drops of chaste tree tincture in water each morning.

- Make an infusion containing equal amounts of raspberry leaf, rosemary, motherwort and gotu kola; drink up to 3 cups daily.

- If tension and stress (*see page* 101) are contributing to loss of libido drink a cup of wood betony and vervain infusion night and morning.

- Take 10 drops of helonias tincture in water three times a day.

- Take up to 600 mg Siberian ginseng and 500 mg evening primrose oil daily.

- Add a few drops of sandalwood or rose oil to bath water before retiring or ask your partner to give you a massage using the same herbs in a little almond oil as a prelude to lovemaking.

Menopause

For most women the menopause passes by with little more inconvenience than occasional hot flushes and night sweats. Periods often stop suddenly without further problem or else gradually fade away in an irregular pattern. For others, the picture is quite different. The menopause can be a time of major emotional upheaval, with depression (*see page* 101), weight gain, and heavy bleeding (*see page* 112). Today, many of these symptoms may be treated by hormone replacement therapy (HRT) which boosts oestrogen levels, although critics still have doubts about the long-term effects of such treatment. For some women (including those with a high risk of osteoporosis) this is a preferred solution, but for those who want to take HRT,

herbal remedies can prove beneficial in both relieving the more troublesome symptoms and helping the body to adjust to new levels of functionality. A healthy lifestyle, with a good diet, regular exercise, a happy and fulfilled outlook and acceptable stress levels is obviously important. Anyone who starts out being depressed, overworked or malnourished is unlikely to pass through the menopause without trauma. Herbalists usually aim to use a hormone-balancing mixture of herbs to help ease the change, although remedies can be helpful to relieve some of the more irritating symptoms. Herbs with a hormonal action include chaste tree, wild yam, helonias and sage, while useful nervines (which soothe and calm the nerves) for emotional stress include skullcap, lemon balm and valerian.

Treatment

- Combine 20 ml/4 tsp each of *He Shou Wu*, vervain, sage, and wild yam with 10 ml/2 tsp each of lavender and liquorice tinctures and take 5 ml/1 tsp three times a day.

- Make an infusion containing equal amounts of motherwort, raspberry leaf, and lady's mantle and take 2 to 3 cups daily; add lime flowers or St John's wort if anxiety (*see page* 101) is a problem.

- Take 10 drops of helonias tincture in water three times a day.

- Take one 200 mg golden seal capsule up to three times a day to help relieve hot flushes.

- Drink a cup of sage infusion up to four times daily to reduce sweating.

- Mix equal amounts of hawthorn flowers and motherwort to make an infusion; drink 2 to 3 cups daily for palpitations (*see page* 91).

- Ease vaginal dryness with creams containing vitamin E and marigold.

Problems in pregnancy

Morning sickness

Morning sickness affects many pregnant women in the first three months but with luck may be limited to a few minutes on rising. In some cases it can last all day and extend through much of the nine months as well. Researchers have found that ginger is extremely effective even in these very severe cases. Up to 1 gm per dose has been used quite safely in hospital trials. Other herbs that can help include fennel, lemon balm, chamomile, helonias and peppermint. They are often best taken in drop doses of tincture.

Treatment

- Mix 10 ml/2 tsp of tinctures of fennel, ginger, lemon balm, chamomile, helonias and peppermint into separate 25 ml/5 tsp dropper bottle and add water. Keep these on the bedside table and put a few drops of any one of them on the tongue before rising. Alternate the remedies as necessary.

- Take two 200 mg of ginger in capsules three times daily. The dose can be increased if necessary, or use crystallized ginger, ginger beer or ginger biscuits if preferred.

- Digestive problems can be a contributing factor; take two 200 mg of slippery elm in capsules three times a day before meals.

Herbs to avoid in pregnancy

Avoid totally in pregnancy:
Aloe
Arbor vitae (*Thuja occidentalis*)
Barberry (*Berberis vulgaris*)
Basil oil
Bugleweed
Chamomile oil
Dang Gui
Devil's claw
Feverfew
Golden seal
Greater celandine (*Chelidonium majus*)
Juniper (*Juniperus communis*)
Lady's mantle
Mistletoe (*Viscum album*)
Motherwort
Mugwort (*Artemisia vulgaris*)
Myrrh
Pennyroyal (*Mentha pulegium*)
Pokeroot (*Phytolacca decandra*)
Rue (*Ruta graveolens*)
Shepherd's purse
Southernwood (*Artemisia abrotanum*)
Tansy (*Tanacetum vulgare*)
Wormwood

Avoid regular high or therapeutic doses:
Angelica (*Angelica archangelica*)
Bitter orange (*Citrus aurentium*)
Cayenne
Celery seed
Cinnamon (*Cinnamomum zeylanicum*)
Cowslip
Elder bark
Fennel
Fenugreek
Garlic
Korean ginseng
Lavender
Marjoram (*Origanum vulgare*)
Parsley
Passion flower
Rhubarb root
Senna (*Senna alexandrina*)
Sage
Thyme oils
Vervain
Wild yam
Yarrow
Yellow dock

Use only in the final stages of pregnancy:
Black cohosh
Blue cohosh
Raspberry
Nutmeg
Wood betony

(Botanical names are only given for those herbs not included in the herb directory in this book.)

Essential oils:
If you are pregnant or breastfeeding do not use essential oils until you have checked with your medical adviser and a trained aromatherapist.

Heartburn, constipation and raised blood pressure

Heartburn in pregnancy can be safely treated with slippery elm or marshmallow. Constipation (*see page* 120) is often exacerbated by the use of supplementary iron tablets, so stay with the gentler remedies – ispaghula or dandelion root – rather than the more powerful anthraquinone laxatives – aloe and rhubarb. Raised blood pressure (*see page* 90) is best treated with an infusion of hawthorn and lime flowers; drink 1 cup three times a day.

Caution: Do not take unnecessary medication during pregnancy and maintain regular contact with health-care professionals, particularly if blood pressure is raised.

Childbirth

Childbirth in Western society can be a clinical affair, with little opportunity for using self-help remedies. Herbs have traditionally been used for all stages of labour and birthing; in the early stages or for home deliveries it is still possible to take some of these helpful and calming teas.

Treatment

- To prepare for childbirth, drink 2 cups of a raspberry leaf infusion every day for the last six weeks of pregnancy. Take an additional 20 drops of blue cohosh tincture in water each day during the final three weeks.

- During the early stages of labour drink an infusion made from equal amounts of wood betony, rose petals and raspberry leaves. During the final stages of labour add an equal amount of basil leaves to the brew and continue sipping.

- Massage the abdomen during the early stages of labour with 10 drops of nutmeg, clove, or sage oil diluted in 15 ml/1 tbsp of almond oil.

- Apply a hot compress soaked in a marigold infusion to the lower abdomen above the pubic area.

- After the birth take homeopathic Arnica 6x tablets every 15–30 minutes for a few hours to help repair stressed tissues.

- During the month following childbirth take a sherry glass of *Dang Gui* tonic wine daily, or use two 200 mg capsules of dried herb daily.

Breastfeeding problems

Breastfeeding has its joys – and also its discomforts. Sore nipples are commonplace and there can be mastitis (when a milk duct becomes blocked and infected), engorgement with excessive milk, or sometimes a lack of milk altogether. Sore nipples are usually caused by poor positioning of the baby who should suck at the whole areola (the dark area around the nipple) rather than just holding on to the nipple itself.

Treatment

- For sore nipples apply marigold and chamomile creams to the areola after each feed.

- A traditional and effective remedy for engorgement is to insert a crushed Savoy cabbage leaf between the bra and the breast; replace every four hours. (A poultice of fresh common plantain leaves is a good alternative to cabbage.) For mastitis you can also make an infusion containing red clover, chamomile, and marigold flowers and drink a cup three or four times a day.

- Excessive milk production can be eased by drinking a cup of sage infusion night and morning. This is also effective in drying up milk at weaning.

- Many herbs will encourage milk flow: make an infusion of fenugreek seeds, fennel, dill, goat's rue, milk thistle and raspberry leaf or vervain or use a combination of these herbs if you prefer the taste; drink a cup night and morning.

Caution: Mastitis may require treatment with antibiotics so always seek professional advice.

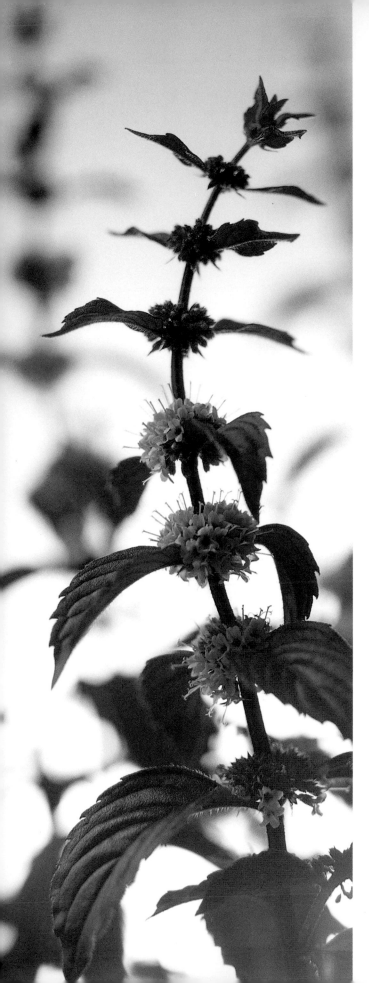

Digestion and liver

Ayurvedic medicine argues that strong digestive fire, or agni, is vital for health in much the same way that medieval physicians warned that 'death dwells in the bowels'. Poor digestive function can lead not only to gastric upsets but also to chronic skin and joint disorders and numerous other health problems. Good diet and healthy function are vital, and many herbs can help to stimulate the digestive organs effectively.

Irritable bowel syndrome

Irritable bowel syndrome (IBS) is a convenient label for a range of symptoms typical of poor digestive function, anxiety or food intolerance. Sufferers usually complain of bloating, flatulence, abdominal pain, and alternating bouts of diarrhoea and constipation (*see page* 120). Stools may contain mucus and blood or else resemble rabbit droppings. Food intolerance is a very common cause: main culprits are dairy food, gluten (found in wheat, oats, barley and rye), caffeine-containing drinks, alcohol, cigarettes, eggs and red meat. Eliminate these from the diet and then gradually reintroduce each one to pinpoint the problem. This is best done with professional guidance. Soothing herbs such as marshmallow, wild yam and meadowsweet can help, and are generally combined with digestive tonics and stimulants like hops, peppermint, vervain, golden seal and milk thistle.

Treatment

- Combine tinctures of wild yam, chamomile, bistort, hops and liquorice. Take 5 ml/1 tsp in a little water three times a day. Add 2–3 drops of peppermint tincture to each dose.

- Drink an infusion of chamomile, vervain and lemon balm three times a day to aid relaxation and reduce gut spasm.

- Use cramp bark tincture to relieve abdominal cramps: take 10 drops in water at 30 minute intervals if symptoms are severe.

- The condition can be linked to the menstrual cycle: take 500–1000 mg of evening primrose or borage (starflower) oil in capsules daily if this is so.

Diverticulosis

Diverticulosis is a problem which usually affects the elderly and often follows a life-long history of constipation and excessive use of laxatives. The problem is caused by a weakening of the muscular wall of the bowel so that small areas of the mucous membrane form pouches, or diverticuli, in which food remnants (particularly pips and seeds) can be trapped, leading to inflammation (diverticulitis). The result is severe cramping pain often accompanied by fever. Around 25 per cent of adults suffer from some degree of diverticulosis in the large intestine and thus run the risk of diverticulitis.

Treatment

- Use ispaghula as a bulking laxative (*see* Constipation, *page* 120).

- Make an infusion of agrimony, hops, red clover and marshmallow leaf. Drink 1 cup three times daily.

- If diverticulitis does develop, take two 200 mg of echinacea or golden seal in capsules three times daily.

- Make a decoction of fenugreek seeds and wild yam and drink three times daily.

- Avoid foods which are likely to produce small, hard residues, such as pips from tomatoes and strawberries. Also avoid fried foods, preserved meats, caffeine and alcohol.

Seek professional help when

- **Vomiting blood or passing blood in the stools.**

- **There is difficulty in swallowing.**

- **There is severe abdominal pain – this needs further investigation.**

- **Diarrhoea persists for more than 36 hours, or for 12 hours or less in young children.**

Gastritis

Gastritis is an inflammation of the stomach lining and is often the result of over-indulgence in rich foods and alcohol. Symptoms include nausea and vomiting (*see page* 122) and diarrhoea (*see page* 121). Chronic gastritis increases the risk of developing stomach or duodenal ulcers, and is often associated with smoking or alcoholism.

Treatment

- Make an infusion of meadowsweet and chamomile and drink a cup up to four times daily.

- Take two 200 mg slippery elm tablets before meals.

- If the gastritis is linked to alcohol abuse take 5 ml/1 tsp of milk thistle tincture in water; repeat every three hours during the day.

- Avoid spices, tea, coffee, alcohol, fried foods and pickles, and eat smaller meals more regularly.

Caution: Gastritis is usually a short-term problems; seek professional help if symptoms persist.

Diet

- Always eat plenty of fibre: fresh vegetables and whole grains rather than wheatbran which can irritate the bowel.

- Remember moderation in all things: not too much alcohol, sweets, sugars, or caffeine-containing drinks.

- Limiting intake of spicy and 'hot' food can be helpful if the digestion is weak.

- Keep to a low-fat, low-meat, low-dairy products regime.

Constipation

Although constipation is extremely common, there is in fact a wide variation in the pattern of bowel motions. Some people think it unusual not to go twice a day while others will be perfectly happy with a motion every third day. Diet is a major contributing factor, with vegetarians and those eating a high-fibre diet likely to have a more frequent pattern of bowel motions than someone eating mainly meat and refined carbohydrates. The food we eat also influences how long it can take to be excreted: for people in the Third World eating a traditional diet, it normally takes around 12 hours or less for food to pass through the gut, whereas for those eating a conventional Western diet it can be as long as 72 hours. A low-fibre diet combined with a lack of exercise – and often coupled with a sluggish lifestyle or personality – lead to what is sometimes called 'flaccid' or 'atonic' constipation. Constipation can also be associated with nervous tension and a hectic lifestyle with little time to respond to the normal urge to defecate (*see* Irritable bowel syndrome, *page* 119). While laxative products are among the best-selling over-the-counter remedies, prolonged use should be avoided: many work by irritating the bowel to encourage movement and over the years such constant irritation leads to weakness and damage with the risk of diverticulosis (*see page* 119).

Treatment

- Atonic constipation can be helped by exercise, a high-fibre diet, and the use of a bulking laxative such as ispaghula: put 1 tsp of seeds into a cup and fill with boiling water. Allow to cool and drink the gelatinous mixture. Flavour with blackcurrant juice to make it more palatable if preferred.

- Constipation associated with tension often responds to bowel relaxants such as chamomile, valerian or wild yam: take a combination of these herbs in tinctures – 5 ml/1 tsp three times a day. If tension is a problem, add an equal amount of cramp bark to the decoction.

- Chinese rhubarb root is a potent laxative – take 10–20 drops of the tincture in water three times a day.

- For general use, make a decoction containing equal amounts of dandelion, yellow dock, liquorice and fennel seeds, and drink a cup three times daily before meals.

- Drink plenty of water – especially a glass of warm water first thing in the morning.

Diarrhoea

Diarrhoea is generally a symptom of imbalance rather than a primary disease, and frequent loose or liquid bowel motions are commonly caused by infection or irritation in the digestive tract. Excessive bowel motions can lead to cramping pains and general soreness in the anal area, while symptoms can include nausea and vomiting. Causes can range from food poisoning and overeating to stress and anxiety. Sudden diarrhoea is most commonly caused by some sort of gastrointestinal infection: this is obvious if others who shared the same meal are similarly affected. Diarrhoea is a common problem for holidaymakers in exotic locations, so never eat raw salads, always wash and peel fruit, and avoid ice cubes in drinks when travelling in areas of dubious hygiene. Diarrhoea and vomiting are the body's natural reaction to an infecting organism and are often the best way of getting rid of it quickly. Regular diarrhoea is more likely to be stress-related. This can range from increased frequency before exams or job interviews to debilitating disorders like ulcerative colitis which require professional help and can lead to chronic illness.

Treatment

- Make a decoction containing equal amounts of bistort and marshmallow. Add a pinch of powdered nutmeg per cup and drink 3 cups a day.

- Combine equal amounts of bistort, agrimony, vervain, and marigold tinctures and add to the holiday first aid kit. Take 10 ml/2 tsp in water up to four times daily as required.

- If nothing else is available, a cup of strong, black, cold Indian tea will effectively ease gut inflammation and soreness.

- Diarrhoea is very dehydrating so increase fluid intake during such bouts. This is especially important for small children who easily become dehydrated.

Caution: Seek professional help if symptoms continue for more than 36 hours, or for more than 12 hours (or less if symptoms are severe) in young children.

Indigestion, acidity, and heartburn

Rushed meals, wearing tight belts, eating irregularly or while feeling tense, or eating too many rich and potentially irritant foods can all contribute to those feelings of heartburn, pain in the lower chest, flatulence and nausea that go under the label of indigestion. Antacids are a popular over-the-counter choice for many, but unfortunately artificially trying to neutralize the normal acid secretions of the stomach often stimulates it to produce even more acid to ensure that the digestion process runs smoothly. Herbal remedies take a rather different approach: relaxing herbs, such as chamomile and lemon balm, will help to reduce the anxiety and tension which can contribute to indigestion, while aromatic carminatives will ease flatulence and nausea (*see pages* 123, 122). Fennel, lemon balm, dill, ginger, galangal, chamomile, and peppermint are all effective. Other herbs, such as meadowsweet and slippery elm, will help to protect the stomach from high acid secretions, while bitter remedies like wormwood and dandelion root will stimulate the digestive process and restore normal function.

Treatment

- Take two 200 mg slippery elm capsules before meals.

- Make an infusion containing equal amounts of cornflower, fennel, and lemon balm. Add a pinch of powdered ginger and 1–2 drops of wormwood tincture to each cup and drink 3 cups daily.

- Drink chamomile, peppermint, or fennel tea after meals.

- Combine meadowsweet, dandelion, and peppermint tinctures and take 20 drops in a little warm water after meals.

Caution: The pain of indigestion can be confused with heart pain from disorders like angina pectoris. This sort of pain eases with rest, while heartburn is generally worse when the sufferer lies down. Sudden severe indigestion in someone who has previously been symptom-free should always be professionally investigated for a possible underlying heart condition. Chronic indigestion can also be a sign of peptic ulcers, gall bladder disorders (*see page* 123), liver problems (*see page* 124), or cancer, and expert diagnosis is essential.

Nausea and vomiting

Nausea and vomiting can be associated with a wide range of illnesses: from life-threatening fevers (*see page* 127) and stomach problems to motion sickness, migraine (*see page* 134) and indigestion (*see page* 121). While many herbs are effective at relieving symptoms, the flavours are not to everyone's taste and they can make symptoms temporarily worse if sufferers really do find them unpleasant.

Treatment

- Ginger is probably the most effective antiemetic (stops vomiting) and is readily available in many forms. Capsules (one to two 200 mg) or tincture (10 drops) are ideal, but crystallized ginger, ginger beer or ginger biscuits may be more palatable for many. Galangal can be used in the same way.

- For nausea associated with stomach upsets combine equal amounts of lemon balm, dandelion and marshmallow tincture and take 20 drops in a little water every 30–60 minutes.

Caution: Seek professional help for severe and persistent problems.

Stomach upsets

Minor stomach upsets with abdominal pain, nausea and vomiting (*see left*), and diarrhoea (*see page* 120) affect most of us at some time. They can often be associated with food poisoning, an excess of rich food or too much alcohol. Chills on the stomach can also cause considerable discomfort. Some people are rather more prone to stomach upsets than others and the problem can be stress-related (*see page* 101), with any increase in nervous tension or anxiety levels (*see page* 101) usually accompanied by digestive problems. Relaxing carminatives such as lemon balm and chamomile can be useful in these cases.

Treatment

- Mix a teaspoon each of powdered slippery elm and marshmallow root, add a little water to make into a paste and swallow. Repeat every three hours if necessary.

- For stomach upsets associated with chills, make a decoction containing ginger or galangal root and cloves. Grate a little nutmeg into each cup and drink 3 cups daily.

- If a nervous tummy is a regular problem, make an infusion combining lemon balm and chamomile and drink a cup every two or three hours while symptoms persist.

Caution: Seek professional advice if symptoms persist for more than 24 hours, and for any severe or unusual abdominal pain.

Preventatives

- Use plenty of garlic in cooking. A low dose is very supportive for the digestion although some find that excessive garlic leads to gastric upsets. One to two cloves daily in a family meal is ideal; reduce this amount if cooking for only one or two.

- Avoid fatty and fried foods and overeating when tired. Drink plenty of water between meals but avoid too much liquid with meals.

- Many traditions focus on balancing foods. In China every meal must contain the right mix of *Yin* and *Yang* foods, to ensure health, while Ayurvedic traditions focus on balancing tastes. In the West, balancing foods, which Galenic medicine classified as 'hot' and 'cold' foods, was part of the standard approach to healthy eating until the 17th century. Cooks would add fennel to fish or pepper to beans to prevent resulting digestive upsets from too much 'cold' or 'damp' foodstuffs.

Flatulence

Wind – whether it goes up or down – is usually more of an embarrassment than an indicator of serious health problems. Adding fennel, dill, rosemary or sage to cooking will often reduce the risk.

Treatment

- Drink peppermint or lemon balm tea after meals.

- Take one 200 mg ginger capsule or 5 drops of ginger or galangal tincture after meals or as necessary.

Candidiasis

There are around 60–70 yeasts which can affect the body although *Candida albicans* is the commonest. These yeasts reside in large numbers in our guts and on the surface of the skin. Like bacteria they usually cause us few problems, but if resistance is weakened by overwork, stress (*see page* 101), or illness, then – being opportunist creatures – they can proliferate and affect our wellbeing. This proliferation not only leads to excessive yeasts in the bowel competing with the other more friendly bacteria which normally live there – thus interfering with digestion – but they may also cause the yeasts to take on a fungal form and be absorbed into the bloodstream, where they can interfere with our own body chemistry and cause a wide variety of health problems. Symptoms can be many and varied, and candidiasis has become something of a catch-all phrase for general, non-specific, health problems.

Treatment

- Make an infusion containing equal amounts of marigold, agrimony, rosemary and echinacea (use the aerial part of *E. purpurea*) and drink a cup three times daily.

- Take garlic supplements – either up to 2 gm of the herb in capsules daily or use two to three cloves in cooking.

- Take 500–1000 mg of evening primrose oil in capsules.

- Avoid yeast-rich foods or those that can encourage yeast growth – sugars, alcohol, dairy products, refined carbohydrates, junk and preserved foods and mycoprotein (protein derived from fungus and mould).

- Eat plenty of 'good bacteria' in the form of *Lactobacillus acidophilus* and *Bifida* spp available in capsules and contained in live yoghurt.

- Supplements of Pau d'Arco capsules (*Tabebuia impetiginosa*), or those containing caprylic acid (a fatty acid that is available as an over-the-counter supplement, and found naturally in breast milk), are also reputed to help.

Gall bladder problems

Bile produced in the liver is stored and concentrated in the gall bladder. The gall bladder can become infected or inflamed and gallstones can be formed if certain substances, such as cholesterol, become particularly concentrated in the bile. Gallstones may be quite symptomless, but if they become large enough to obstruct the gall duct they can lead to jaundice and severe pain. Heartburn (*see page* 121) after eating fatty meals often suggests that the gall bladder is not working as efficiently as it should. Many herbs – known as cholagogues – will stimulate bile flow and normalize gall bladder function. They include golden seal, rosemary, sage, boneset, yellow dock, fringe tree and dandelion.

Treatment

- Make a decoction of equal amounts of fringe tree, dandelion and milk thistle. Add 2–3 drops of wormwood tincture to each cup and drink up to 3 cups daily.

- Combine wild yam, milk thistle and echinacea tinctures and take 5 ml/1 tsp three times daily in water.

- Avoid fatty foods and dairy products.

Caution: Gall bladder problems need professional support and treatment. Use self-help remedies only in mild cases, or stable cases where the diagnosis is certain.

Liver problems

The liver is the largest organ in the body and is often described as its chemical factory: processing fatty acids, producing essential enzymes, storing nutrients and maintaining the quality of the blood. It is also in the front line of the body's defences as it breaks down the various chemicals absorbed in digestion and prevents harmful substances reaching the circulation and brain. In our polluted world, the liver is thus under considerable stress to ensure that only safe and familiar substances are absorbed into the body. It is hardly surprising, then, that this overworked organ can become a little sluggish, leading to digestive problems. Many herbs have a cleansing and stimulating effect on the liver, so while liver disorders in general require expert treatment, several herbs are liver tonics which can support orthodox treatment or help to improve function. Other herbs will help to repair cells and restore normal function – these include milk thistle seeds or dandelion root. Bitter herbs and foods generally act as liver stimulants. These include globe artichoke, chicory, dandelion root, wormwood, chicory hops, white horehound and gotu kola.

Treatment

- As a general liver tonic, combine dandelion, burdock and milk thistle in a decoction and drink 1 cup every day.

- Make an infusion of vervain, agrimony and lemon balm and drink 3 cups daily.

- In chronic conditions, drink a decoction of milk thistle, fringe tree and yellow dock three times daily to support additional professional treatment.

- A decoction of dandelion root or an infusion of vervain tea after meals will help maintain normal function.

Caution: Professional treatment and regular liver function tests are essential: do not depend on self-help remedies.

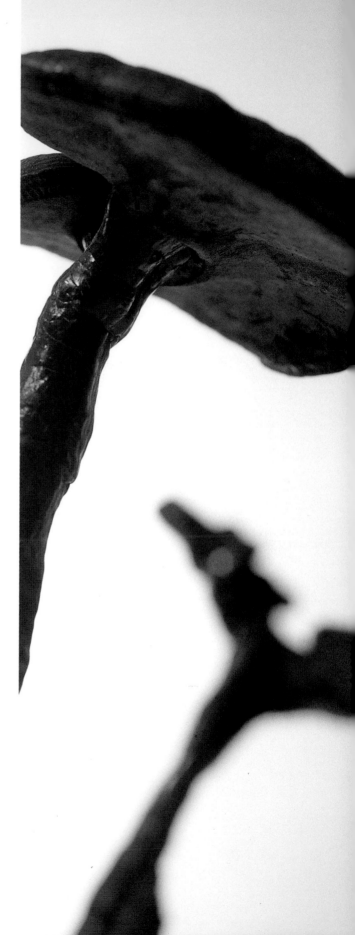

Infections

Long before science discovered the bacteria and viruses which cause infections, herbs were being used to repel the 'venoms' or 'evils' which earlier generations blamed for ill health. We now know that many of these plants have antibiotic properties. Faced with infection, the body's immune system goes into battle, raising the temperature and increasing the production of white blood cells. Herbs can be used to strengthen the immune response rather than suppress the symptoms.

Fevers

High temperature is part of the body's normal response to fighting infection. In traditional fever management the aim is to cool the body as the temperature soars and warm during the 'shivering' phase. During the 'hot' stage herbs such as yarrow, lime flowers or boneset can be used to encourage sweating, while bitter herbs such as white horehound or wormwood can stimulate digestion; during the 'chill' stage of the fever, herbal stimulants like nutmeg, cloves, ginger or galangal can alternately heat the system.

Treatment

- Make an infusion containing equal amounts of catmint, vervain and boneset and drink a cup during the hot stages.

- During the chill stage drink a cup of decoction made from a couple of slices of ginger or galangal root with two cloves.

- Take 5–10 ml/1–2 tsp of echinacea tincture in water every three hours to combat infection.

- Use a compress soaked in lavender or marigold infusion to cool a fevered forehead during the hot phase and sponge the body with the same mixture. In the chill stage use rosemary or basil infusion in the same way.

Caution: High fevers require skilled treatment so confine home remedies to milder cases and seek professional help whenever temperatures reach 39°C/102.2°F for more than a couple of hours.

Seek professional help when

- **Fever and high temperatures (39°C/102.2°F) last for more than a couple of hours and do not respond to treatment.**

- **There is severe pain in the respiratory tract or chest pain.**

- **Symptoms of colds and flu are accompanied by a rash or neck stiffness.**

- **Shingles is severe, especially if facial nerves are affected.**

The common cold

Colds are caused by a viral infection, with symptoms likely to include sore throats, blocked noses and coughs and sneezes. Viruses regularly mutate so repeated infections can be common, especially where sufferers are run-down or overtired. Traditionally colds were associated with some sort of external factor, such as cold weather or getting soaked in a rainstorm. Modern medicine may dismiss these causes in favour of viruses but we are certainly more susceptible to colds if we are tired, overworked, unhappy or have been abnormally chilled by the extremes of climate. Because colds are caused by a virus they cannot be treated by antibiotics which are only good for tackling bacteria. Some herbs do possess antiviral activity and so are ideal, while the herbal approach also focuses on strengthening the body's immune system. Echinacea is one of the best herbs to take to strengthen the immune system and garlic is especially helpful if the cold develops into a chest infection. Anticatarrhals such as elder flower and yarrow can ease the symptoms.

Preventatives

- Take plenty of exercise, fresh air, and sunlight. Learn to relax – yoga, *Tai Ch'i Chuan*, or *Qi Gong* classes are all suitable.

- Avoid becoming overtired or overstressed: if your workload is a problem then it may be time to reassess your lifestyle. To combat short-term stresses take up to 600 mg of Siberian ginseng daily for up to four weeks.

- A daily garlic supplement (up to 2 gm a day or equivalent) can be taken long term (for three months or more).

- Take three 200 mg capsules (or 10 ml/2 tsp of tincture) of echinacea or *Huang Qi* daily to boost the immune system for up to four weeks.

Treatment:

- Make an infusion using 1 tsp of dried hemp agrimony to a cup of boiling water. Add the juice of 1 lemon, 1 tsp of grated fresh ginger and 1 tsp of honey. Drink a cup three to four times daily.

- Add 10 drops of eucalyptus oil and 5 drops of peppermint oil to a basin of boiling water as a steam inhalation.

- At the first sign of symptoms take up to 10 ml/2 tsp of echinacea tincture in water or three 200 mg echinacea capsules three times daily for up to five days.

- Cut down on refined carbohydrates (sugar and white flour products) as these tend to encourage mucus, and eat plenty of fruit instead.

- Taking up to 5 gm of vitamin C a day (short-term use only) can also help.

- Ease any particularly severe symptoms with appropriate remedies (*see* Sore throats, *page* 97, Catarrh, *page* 96, Coughs, *page* 96, Fevers, *page* 127).

- Follow the regimes suggested for Recurrent infections (*page* 127) if persistent colds are a problem.

Influenza

Influenza is a viral infection so it will not respond to antibiotic treatment. It is characterized by all the symptoms of a severe cold (*see page* 126), as well as headaches, painful muscles, weakness and high temperature. An attack typically lasts for about a week but it will often leave the sufferer feeling depressed and debilitated for several weeks. Herbal remedies are similar to those used for the common cold, with particular emphasis on plants like boneset, garlic, ginger, lavender and elder.

Treatment:

• Make an infusion by combining 1 tsp each of dried boneset, echinacea leaves (*E. purpurea*), elder flowers, lavender flowers and peppermint to ¹/₂ litre/1 pint of boiling water. Drink 1 cup up to six times a day, reheating as required.

• Take up to 2 gm of garlic in capsules daily.

• Ease any particularly severe symptoms with appropriate remedies (*see* Headaches, *page* 134, Sore throats, *page* 97, Catarrh, *page* 96, Coughs, *page* 96, Fevers, *page* 127).

• To combat lingering debility and coughs simmer 2 tsp of elecampane root and 2 tsp of wild oat straw (use whole grains if oat straw is not available) in ¹/₂ litre/1 pint of water for 15 minutes and drink a cup night and morning.

• Use a compress soaked in lavender or marigold infusion to ease feverish headaches.

• Drink an infusion of St John's wort and lemon balm up to three times a day if depression (*see page* 101) is a problem in the weeks following a bad attack.

Recurrent infections

Persistent colds, crops of boils, chronic fatigue or repeated urinary infections (*see pages* 126, 128, 104, 114) can often indicate a reduced resistance to infection, and because the immune system may been weakened by stress, overwork or food allergies, it is harder for it to combat bacteria, viruses and fungi. Such organisms are extremely opportunistic and can very rapidly get out of hand. Many tonic herbs have a reputation for strengthening the immune system and anyone feeling run down or suffering constant minor infections may benefit. A number of traditional Chinese tonics can also boost the immune system and some are becoming available in the West: *Huang Qi* and reishi can be very effective and it is well worth using shiitake mushrooms in cooking as they also have a similar immune enhancing effect.

Treatment

• Take up to 600 mg daily of echinacea in capsules or tablets for up to three weeks.

• Drink the fresh juice of 1 lemon in a glass of hot water with 1 tsp of honey each morning.

• Combine 10 drops each of eucalyptus, thyme and lavender oil with 25 ml/5 tsp of almond oil, and ask your partner to massage your chest and back every evening.

• Make a tonic wine by soaking 250 mg of *Huang Qi* root in a bottle of red wine (ensuring that the herb is well covered) for two weeks. Strain the mix and drink a sherry glass daily.

• Use plenty of garlic in cooking or take 2 gm a day in capsules.

Boils and carbuncles

A skin inflammation containing pus is generally caused by a staphylococcal infection of a hair follicle. Boils often arise because of reduced resistance to infection – perhaps due to exhaustion, overwork or chronic illness. There could also be some deep-seated septic focus – such as a dental abscess adding to the overall toxicity. A cluster of boils is known as a carbuncle; treatment can include the use of poultices or drawing ointments – often based on slippery elm – to encourage the boil to discharge, combined with herbs to boost the immune system and combat bacterial infections.

Supplements

- For colds, flu or recurrent infections take up to 5 gm of vitamin C daily for up to one week. Reduce the dosage if there are digestive upsets or diarrhoea.

- Take a zinc supplement to boost the immune system: studies suggest up to 50 mg daily can help combat colds and infections, although for long-term use 20–30 mg a day (5–10 mg for children) is more normal.

- Ensure a good supply of essential fatty acids: take 5 ml/1 tsp daily of walnut, safflower or pumpkin oil or 250 mg of evening primrose or borage (starflower) oil if persistent infections are a problem.

- Take a vitamin B complex supplement: choose one that is not yeast-based and delivers no more than 10 mg daily of vitamin B_6.

Treatment

- Apply a drawing ointment made from garlic, slippery elm or chickweed three to four times a day to encourage the boil to discharge its pus. Then use an antibacterial cream – echinacea, marigold or tea tree – two to three times a day.

- Take two 200 mg echinacea to boost the immune system.

- Take up to 600 mg of Siberian ginseng daily if stress (*see page* 101) is contributing to the problem.

- Follow the regimes suggested for Recurrent infections (*see page* 127) if repeated outbreaks of boils occur.

Caution: Recurrent or persistent boils can indicate diabetes or kidney problems. Unskilled lancing of boils can spread infection and is best avoided.

Cold sores

These are recurrent, localized sores caused by the *Herpes simplex* virus which is carried by around 50 per cent of the adult population. The sores take the form of tiny blisters which usually start with a tingling sensation and rapidly develop into inflamed, red areas occurring around the mouth, but they are sometimes found elsewhere on the body. Once a person has been infected, the virus can remain dormant in the body for years, usually causing a recurrent outbreak of cold sores if the sufferer is at all rundown or overtired. The virus is extremely contagious during the blistering stage. Cold sores are more of a nuisance than a serious health hazard. They will respond well to herbs, although it is best to start treatment as soon as the familiar tingling sensation starts.

Treatment:

- Simmer 2 slices of fresh ginger in 1 cup of water for ten minutes. Process fresh cleavers in a food processor and strain to produce 30 ml/2 tbsp of juice. Combine the decoction and cleavers juice with the juice of half a lemon and drink the mixture one or two times a day.

- Boost the immune system with remedies suggested under Recurrent infections (*see page* 127)

- Apply 1–2 drops of 50 per cent lavender or tea tree oil directly to the sore when the warning tingling first starts.

- Use echinacea or marigold cream on the sore once blisters have appeared.

Shingles

Like chickenpox, shingles is caused by the *Herpes zoster* virus. Typically it starts with pain and a red, blistering rash along the route of a nerve (such as across the face or chest). Symptoms usually ease within about three weeks, although severe pain along the affected nerve can persist for months. Recent research has shown that powdered cayenne can be very effective to ease this – add it to creams or make a hot infused oil. During an attack, echinacea will help to combat the viral infection while drinking plenty of St John's wort infusion can help to limit the risk of lingering nerve pain so commonly associated with shingles.

Treatment:

- Make a decoction of 4 tsp of echinacea root to 2 cups of water and combine with an infusion of 2 tsp St John's wort to 2 cups of water. Drink a cup of the combined mixture three to four times daily.

- Apply the fresh juice of aloe vera leaves to the rash three to four times a day. Alternatively, use 1 tsp of powdered slippery elm made into a paste with a little water or milk and apply to the rash; cover with a clean gauze if necessary.

- Make an infusion containing equal amounts of passion flower and lemon balm to ease pain and combat the infection.

- Lingering pain can be eased by applying cayenne infused oil or ointment. Add 50 g/2 oz of chopped chili to 250 ml /8 fl oz of sunflower oil. Alternatively, use vervain or St John's wort in creams or infused oils.

Caution: Professional treatment is advised in severe cases, or where facial nerves (for example around the eyes) are involved.

Diet

- Cut down on refined carbohydrates (sugar and white flour products) as these tend to lead to a build up of mucus which can encourage infection. If you have persistent infections or are suffering from colds or flu cut out these foods completely.

- While fruit is a good food to combat infection, too much fructose is not: eat no more than four pieces of fruit a day.

- Avoid potentially harmful stimulants such as tea, coffee and chocolate, as well as tobacco and alcohol.

- Masked food allergies can weaken the immune system: if bowel disturbances, vague aches and pains, or migraine (*see page* 134) are also common symptoms, then consider an exclusion diet or cut out the commonest allergens (such as milk, wheat, gluten, or beef) for at least three weeks to see if the condition improves.

- Persistent use of antibiotics can also weaken the immune system, so try to avoid taking too many and seek alternatives, especially for children.

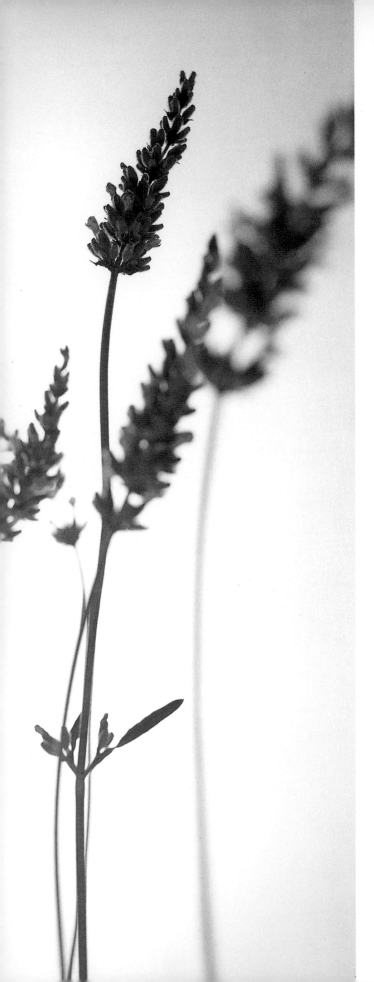

Aches and pains

Aching muscles or creaking joints usually send sufferers reaching for painkillers; while these might relieve the symptoms they do little to encourage healing or treat the cause of the problem. Herbal remedies can help do both – and ease some of the discomfort as well. Long-term aches, such as arthritis or gout, often respond to dietary changes, with herbs used as cleansing remedies to clear toxins from the system.

Arthritis

Arthritis simply means an inflammation of a joint, but there are various types, each requiring rather different treatment, so it is important to be sure of the exact diagnosis. Osteoarthritis is the wear and tear variety that afflicts more than half of the population as we grow older. Rheumatoid arthritis is a more serious and potentially crippling disease. While osteoarthritis tends to affect only a few of the body's joints, rheumatoid arthritis can affect many of them. This sort of arthritis is an inflammatory problem and can be related to a variety of hereditary health problems. Women are three times more likely than men to develop rheumatoid arthritis. Arthritis can also occur in children and always needs professional medical treatment. Arthritis may be related to food intolerance, so eliminating possible allergens such as dairy products, wheat, gluten, beef or pork can be worth trying in chronic conditions.

Treatment

- Combine equal amounts of tinctures of St John's wort, white willow, celery, black cohosh and yellow dock. Take 5 ml/1 tsp in warm water four times a day.

- Localized osteoarthritis can respond to topical, long-term treatment: apply a comfrey cream or infused oil every night and morning for at least two months.

- Herbalists call osteoarthritis a 'cold' condition that is often eased by heat. Add 10 drops of a warming oil like rosemary to 5 ml/1 tsp of infused comfrey oil and massage the aching joint every 30–60 minutes. Alternatively, make an infused cayenne oil and use that; dilute with more almond oil if this causes skin irritation.

- Make an infusion of equal parts meadowsweet, boneset and yarrow and take three times a day to encourage sweating, which will help to clear toxins.

- Devil's claw tablets are a valuable addition to treatment – take two 200 mg capsules of the herb three to four times daily; maintain this dose for at least six weeks.

- Put a mixture of 50 g/1¾ oz of Epsom salts and 10 drops of rosemary into the bath water at night.

- Calcium supplements may also be helpful, especially among postmenopausal (*see* Menopause, *page* 115) women.

- Many people find feverfew helpful – take one 200 mg capsule three times daily; stop treatment if mouth ulcers result.

- For rheumatoid arthritis make an infusion of celery and St John's wort tea and drink up to 4 cups a day.

Caution: Rheumatoid arthritis always needs professional treatment; only use self-help remedies to support orthodox treatment.

Rheumatism and fibrositis

Rheumatism is a very non-precise term that is used to describe the various aches and pains suffered in joints or muscles, and may be referred to as myalgia, which simply means pain in the muscles. Fibrositis is an inflammation of fibrous tissue, which leads to pain and stiffness and can be treated with anti-inflammatories and those remedies recommended for rheumatic disorders. Orthodox medicine will generally prescribe painkillers, while the herbal approach will usually involve the use of cleansing herbs to remove any chemical toxins that are lingering in the tissues. Diuretics, digestive stimulants, circulatory stimulants and laxatives are all likely to be found in herbal remedies for rheumatism.

Treatment

- Make an infusion combining equal amounts of meadowsweet, yarrow and rosemary, and drink a cup three times a day.

Seek professional help when

- **Headaches are severe or recurrent and persist for more than 48 hours without responding to treatment.**

- **Sprains or strains are accompanied by severe bruising – there may be a fracture or cracked bone.**

- **There is severe pain or any loss of sensation or movement.**

- Use 20 ml/4 tsp of infused oil of bladderwrack with 5 drops each of lavender, thyme and eucalyptus oils on aching areas several times a day.

- Warm compresses can sometimes help: soak a pad in a mixture of 10 ml/2 tsp arnica tincture, 20 ml/4 tsp cramp bark and 20 ml/4 tsp black cohosh tincture with 150 ml/5 fl oz of hot water, and apply to the painful area. Reheat the mixture for a fresh compress. Do not use arnica on broken skin.

Backache, lumbago and sciatica

Backache is one of the most common causes for taking days off work, and visiting the doctor or seeking alternative medical treatment. Causes range from pulled muscles and damaged discs (the spongy plugs that separate the vertebrae and act as shock absorbers), to poor posture, kidney disease, gynaecological problems or simply sitting in an awkward position for long periods. Lumbago means pain in the lower back (the lumbar region) from whatever cause, whereas sciatica is technically a pain felt along the back and outer side of the thigh, leg and foot, with accompanying back pain and stiffness usually involving the sciatic nerve. If mechanical damage is involved, then manipulative therapies like osteopathy may be necessary to solve the problem.

Supplements and diet

- Avoiding refined carbohydrates (white sugar and flour) as well as cutting down on red meat, shellfish, alcohol, caffeine, dairy products and tomatoes, potatoes and peppers (all members of the nightshade family) can often be helpful for those suffering from arthritic or rheumatic disorders.

- Take additional B and E vitamins for arthritic problems. Calcium and beta-carotene supplements may also help.

- Many ready-made rubs are available over-the-counter – look for mixtures containing juniper, cajeput (*Melaleuca leucadendron*), wintergreen, birch, pine or camphor oils as well as the oils listed in the remedies above.

For persistent backache with no obvious cause, changing sleeping arrangements can sometimes help: a firm mattress is essential – although firm here means supportive rather than hard. Alternatively, lying on your back with your knees bent or curling into a small ball with the spine curved in the foetal position as you fall asleep, can also bring relief.

Treatment

- Make a massage rub containing 20 drops each of lavender, thyme and eucalyptus oils in 20 ml/4 tsp of infused St John's wort oil. Ask a friend or partner to massage it gently into the aching area of the back night and morning.

- A compress soaked in 15 ml/1 tbsp of cramp tincture and 5 ml/1 tsp of ginger tincture diluted with 100 ml/4 fl oz of hot water can help relieve painful sprains and backaches.

- Take a mixture of St John's wort, cramp and white willow tinctures in warm water.

- Drink an infusion of St John's wort and wood betony if the pain is bad.

- If the pain starts with an accidental injury then take homeopathic Arnica 6x tablets immediately and repeat at hourly intervals for up to 12 hours to ease shock and trauma.

Caution: Massage is not appropriate if there is inflammation or any kind of injury: seek professional advice if in doubt. If sudden back pain does not clear or ease within three or four days, seek professional help.

Frozen shoulder and tennis elbow

These common problems are usually treated by corticosteroid injections. Frozen shoulder is a chronic stiffness of the shoulder joint, usually with no obvious cause, while tennis elbow involves inflammation of the tendons and usually follows excessive use of the forearm muscles. Frozen shoulder can be related to stress (*see page* 101) and tension and a suppressed desire to 'hit out' at whatever is causing the problem.

Treatment

- Make a rub containing 5 ml/1 tsp each of lavender and yarrow or chamomile oils in 40 ml/8 tsp of St John's wort oil. Massage the affected areas frequently.

Cramp

The severe pain of cramp is caused by a sudden contraction of the muscles; commonly this occurs in calf muscles, which become hard and tense. Rubbing the muscle vigorously can bring rapid relief. Cramp can be caused by unaccustomed exercise, stress, tiredness, or poor posture, or there might be an imbalance of the salts in the body, especially in hot weather. Cramp is common in pregnancy. Herbal massage oils can be helpful and internal remedies containing wild yam or cramp bark can help relax muscles.

Treatment

- Make a rub by adding 40 drops of lavender oil and 40 drops of chamomile oil to 25 ml/5 tsp of cramp bark tincture and 20 ml/4 tsp of almond oil. Shake the mixture very thoroughly and massage a little into the affected areas. Repeat as required.

- Stimulate the circulation with galangal or ginger tea two or three times a day and take garlic and vitamin C supplements regularly.

- Take 40 drops of cramp bark tincture three times a day if the problem is persistent.

- For cramps in the legs at night – often associated with varicose veins – try 20–40 drops of melilot tincture in half a tumbler of warm water before retiring.

- Supplements of vitamins B and D, calcium tablets, and an adequate salt intake can also help.

- In hot climates salt tablets can be useful for those prone to cramps.

Gout

The severe pain and swelling associated with gout are caused by a build up of uric acid crystals in the joints – commonly the big toe joint; this is associated with an inability to break down a group of chemicals called purines that are found in shellfish, fatty fish, red meat and offal. Cutting out these foods and caffeine and smoking can help. Herbal treatment focuses on clearing the toxins.

Treatment

- Make an infusion combining equal amounts of celery seed, yarrow and meadowsweet and drink a cup three times daily.

- Alternatively, brew a decoction of black cohosh, white willow and celery seeds and drink a cup three times daily.

- Apply a mixture of 5 drops of clove oil in 5 ml/1 tsp of almond oil to the affected area or soak a compress in 10 drops of clove oil in 100 ml/4 fl oz of warm water.

- Use mashed cabbage leaf as a poultice: place it gently on the affected area, if the sufferer can tolerate it.

- Asparagus is a good diuretic and can be helpful – eat plenty when in season.

- Devil's claw tablets are an effective anti-inflammatory and may be useful – take two 200 mg capsules of the herb three to four times daily.

- Oxalic acid is another food residue that can build up in the joints, so also avoid rhubarb, sorrel and spinach.

Sprains and strains

Pulled muscles and twisted joints can be acutely painful, and if they are the result of some accidental, traumatic injury then an X-ray may be necessary to identify fractures. Strains involve a slight tearing of a muscle or the tendon attaching it to a bone and are usually caused by overstretching. Sprains are a tear in the joint capsule or associated ligaments and are caused by twisting.

Treatment

- Arnica is the ideal remedy for any damaged tissues. Apply a little cream several times a day or use a compress soaked in 10 ml/2 tsp of arnica tincture to 200 ml/7 fl oz of hot water. Do not use arnica if the skin is broken. Take homeopathic Arnica 6x every four hours after painful and accidental sprains and strains.

- Use elastic or tubular bandages to support the injured joint or limb where possible.

- Make a rub containing 5 drops each of rosemary, thyme, sage and lavender oils in an infused comfrey oil base and apply night and morning.

Headaches and migraine

Headaches are usually a symptom of some underlying disorder rather than a primary illness. Causes are numerous and the location and character of the pain is often an indication of the problem: pains centred behind the eyes can suggest an underlying digestive disturbance; those starting at the back of the neck and creeping forward are often tension headaches; pains and sensitivity around the eyes or above the nose can be caused by a sinus problem (*see page* 97). Migraine is typically preceded by visual disturbances and increased sensitivity to light. Attacks can often be related to food intolerance, so identifying the cause is important: red wine, chocolate, pork, citrus fruits, coffee and cheese are all common culprits.

Treatment

- For common headaches with no apparent cause mix equal amounts of wood betony, St John's wort and passion flower and drink a cup every two hours until the pain eases.

- Massage a mixture of 20 drops of lavender oil in 10 ml/2 tsp sweet almond oil into the nape of neck and temples at the first signs of a migraine (normally the preliminary visual disturbance phase).

- Drink a cup of lavender infusion if the headache is eased by a cold compress to the head, or a cup of rosemary infusion if it responds better to a hot towel on the forehead.

- Many migraine sufferers find that chewing fresh feverfew leaves can help to prevent attacks. However, the fresh plant can cause mouth ulcers in sensitive individuals, so it should not be taken if this side effect develops.

Caution: Seek professional help for any severe or recurrent headache which persists for more than 48 hours and does not respond to treatment.

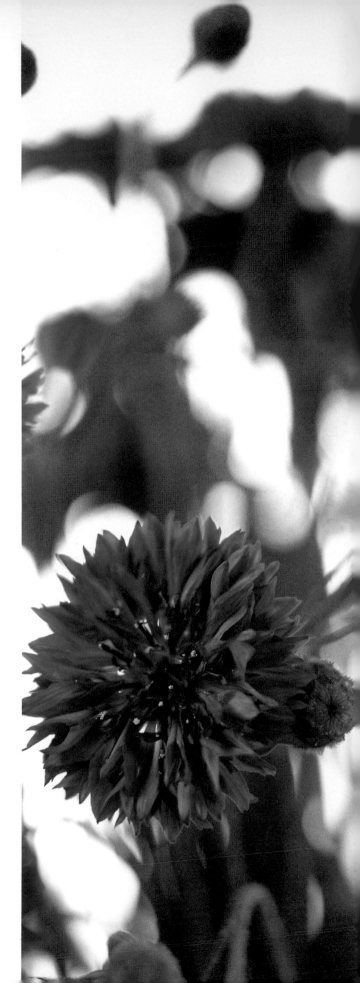

Eyes

Our eyes are in constant use: transmitting images of what is around us to the brain while coping with closely placed computer screens, the dust and grit of city streets and overbright sunshine, thanks to ozone depletion. Yet we take our eyes almost totally for granted. Regular eye exercises – alternately focusing on near and distant objects, or splashing with cold water each morning – can help keep them working well.

Conjunctivitis

Conjunctivitis – commonly known as 'red eye' – is an inflammation of the mucous membrane covering the eyeball. It is usually caused by an infection although conjunctivitis can also be associated with dusty, polluted air or a drying of the eye's normal secretions in old age. Sufferers generally complain of discomfort, watering and a 'gritty feeling' on blinking. Herbs such as eyebright and marigold can be used to bathe and soothe the eye.

Treatment

- Apply moistened tea bags of Indian or Chinese tea, fennel or chamomile to the eyes as a poultice and relax for 15 minutes.

- Use infusions of eyebright, marigold, chamomile, fennel, rose petals or raspberry leaf in eyebaths.

- Take up to 2 gm of garlic in capsules daily to combat infection.

Caution: If the condition has not cleared within three days seek professional advice.

Seek professional help when

- **Symptoms of conjunctivitis continue for more than three days.**

- **There is visual distortion, such as seeing haloes around lights at night.**

- **Regular eyestrain and headaches suggest poor vision – take an eye test as you may need spectacles.**

- **There is a history of glaucoma (raised eyeball pressure) in the family; regular check-ups are needed.**

Herbal eyebaths

Diluted herb tinctures or weak infusions can be very soothing for a range of eye complaints and are simple to use. The mixtures should not sting at all – if they do, dilute further as individual sensitivity can vary.

Make a decoction of your chosen herb using, in most cases, 15 g/½ oz of dried herb to 600 ml/20 fl oz of water reduced to about 400 ml/14 fl oz. Simmer for 10–15 minutes to ensure sterility and then strain well through a fine tea strainer or sieve. Ensure that there are no particles of herb remaining which might irritate the eye.

Allow the mixture to cool to a lukewarm temperature and then fill an eyebath with the mixture. Bathe the eye by placing the eyebath over the eye, lean back so that the eye is well wetted, and blink several times. If both eyes are affected then either use a fresh eyebath or thoroughly clean the first eyebath with boiling water before repeating for the second eye. This is especially important for infectious conditions where cross-contamination is a common problem.

Alternatively, add 2 drops of tincture to an eyebath filled with freshly boiled water which has been allowed to cool.

Bathe the eye at least once a day or when needed, to reduce pain and inflammation.

Useful eyebaths

Conjunctivitis and blepharitis: Eyebright, agrimony, fennel, pot marigold, elder flower, chamomile.

Eye strain/tired eyes: Cornflower, eyebright, raspberry leaf, pot marigold, mullein, chamomile.

Arc eye (caused by exposure to bright light as in welding) and other painful inflammations: Self-heal, eyebright, pot marigold, elder flower.

Hay fever (*see page* 97): Eyebright, agrimony, raspberry leaf, pot marigold, chamomile.

Blepharitis

This is an inflammation of the eyelid. It can be caused by an allergic reaction to cosmetics and is often accompanied by white scales on the lashes. In chronic cases the eyelid can become ulcerated with a yellow crust, and the eyelashes are often matted and may fall out. Blepharitis is common in children following infections like measles (*see page* 150).

Treatment

- Drink a cup of an infusion containing equal amounts of vervain, yarrow and wood betony three times a day to combat the stress caused by the irritation.

- Take one to two 200 mg of echinacea in tablets three times daily.

- Apply fresh aloe vera sap directly to the affected area. Slices of raw potato will also bring relief.

- Marigold or chickweed cream can be applied directly to the affected area.

- Use chamomile, fennel, red clover, raspberry leaf or elder flower infusion in an eyebath.

Styes

A stye is an acute inflammation of the glands responsible for lubricating the eyelashes. Symptoms include redness and swelling of the eyelid and a yellow abscess at the eyelash root. Like cold sores (*see page* 128), styes are generally a sign that the sufferer is rundown – this lowered resistance is usually due to stress (*see page* 101), overwork or recurrent infections (*see page* 127). Rest, relaxation and a good diet are just as important as topical treatments.

Treatment
- Apply a little marigold cream or fresh aloe vera sap to the affected area. Repeat four or five times a day. Evening primrose oil may also be helpful.

- Apply used chamomile or fennel tea bags as a poultice and relax for 15 minutes.

- Take up to 2 gm of garlic or six 200 mg of echinacea in capsules daily.

- If the condition is related to stress, use some of the relaxing teas and anti-stress remedies given on page 101.

Tired eyes and eyestrain

Long working days in artificial or especially bright or dim light, long periods of reading and doing close work, especially in front of a computer screen, incorrectly prescribed glasses, watching television for lengthy periods in the dark, pollution, and day-to-day stresses all combine to make eyestrain a common problem. When it occurs, there may be a feeling of tightness around the eyes, difficulties in focusing, and headaches. Prevention is simple: make sure that there is good light on the page and take brief rest breaks every hour from the computer screen or close work and focus on distant objects for a few seconds. Have your eyes checked – be sure to wear the glasses you are prescribed – and do not watch television in the dark. Closing your eyes and pressing very gently on the eyelids with your palms can also help, if you wear contact lenses, take them out first. In traditional Chinese medicine the eyes are associated with the liver and discomfort can often follow overindulgence or too much rich food.

Treatment
- A simple remedy is to lie down in a darkened room, place slices of cucumber over the eyelids, and relax for ten minutes.

- Make an infusion containing equal amounts of *Ju Hua*, wood betony and gotu kola with a pinch of peppermint. Drink a cup three or four times a day.

- Bathe the eyes in an infusion of cornflower or use any of the eyebaths suggested left.

Supplements

- Take up to 500 mg of vitamin C daily, as well as low doses of vitamin A or beta-carotene. Eating carrots and dark green leafy vegetables will also boost beta-carotene intake.

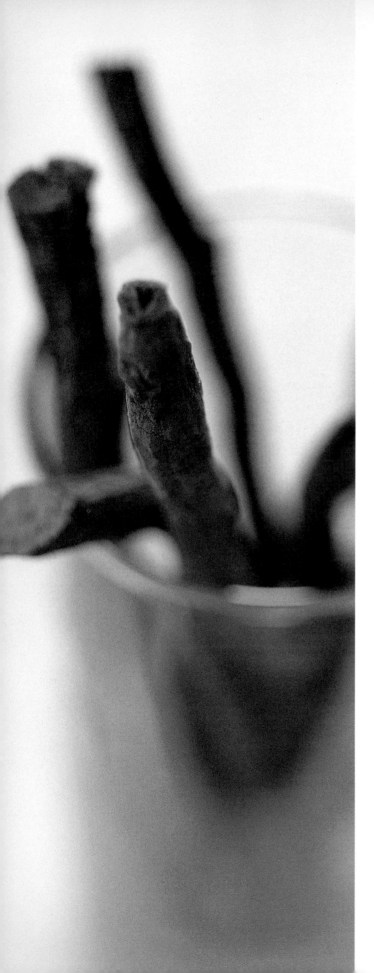

Glands

The body's endocrine system includes
the pituitary, thyroid, and adrenal glands,
ovaries, testes, and parts of the pancreas. These
glands are responsible for producing a variety of
hormones, and dysfunction soon upsets body
chemistry. There are also exocrine glands which
produce secretions like saliva and sometimes these
too can cause health problems. The lymphatic
system, which transports various fluids around the
body, also contains a number of nodes which are
popularly referred to as 'glands', although they are
really quite different organs. Herbs are useful for
both endocrine and exocrine glands, as they
influence body chemistry to normalize production
of particular hormones and enzymes as well as
combat infections and inflammations.

Late-onset diabetes

Diabetes is associated with a failure by the pancreas to produce sufficient insulin to break down the sugars in our food. Juvenile onset is often hereditary and leads to insulin-dependence, but the late-onset variety – usually starting in the 60s or 70s – is an all-too-common result of a lifetime of poor diet with too many sugars and an irregular pattern of meals. Many herbs are hypoglycaemic (they will reduce blood sugar levels), while others are hyperglycaemic (they will help to raise levels for those with low blood sugar). Late-onset diabetics are usually given blood or urine testing kits to maintain regular monitoring of their blood sugar levels. Herbal teas can help reduce high levels but their use does need care and regular monitoring.

Treatment

- Make an infusion from equal amounts of fenugreek seeds, bilberry leaves, stinging nettles and goat's rue. Drink a cup two or three times daily.

- Take two 200 mg of fenugreek in capsules twice a day.

- Take 10 ml/2 tsp of aloe vera juice daily.

- Use plenty of garlic in cooking or take up to 2 gm daily in capsules.

- Take 10 drops of fringe tree bark tincture in water three times a day.

- Eat a diet rich in complex carbohydrates and fibre, such as brown rice, whole grains, oats, beans and vegetables.

- Banana, papaya, cabbage, lettuce, turnip and olives will all encourage insulin production.

Cautions: Insulin-dependent diabetics should not take hypoglycaemic herbs unless under professional guidance. Late-onset diabetics should consult their health-care professional before attempting self-help remedies.

Glandular fever

Thought to be caused by the Epstein-Barr virus, glandular fever (infectious mononucleosis) is typified by enlarged and tender lymph nodes in the neck, armpits and groin, with loss of appetite, headache (*see page 134*), fever (*see page* 127), sore throat (*see page 97*) and general lethargy. There is a long incubation period and symptoms may persist for several weeks, often leaving sufferers drained and debilitated. The syndrome is especially common in young adults.

Treatment

- Make a decoction of 25 g/1 oz of echinacea root to ½ litre/ 1 pint of water. Process enough fresh cleavers in a food processor to make 30 ml/2 tbsp juice when strained. Combine the juice with a pinch of powdered dried chili, the juice of half a lemon and enough echinacea decoction to make up to 1 cup. Drink 1 cup every three to four hours.

- Take two 200 mg garlic capsules at night.

- Once symptoms ease, make a tea by decocting 2 tsp of elecampane root in ½ litre/1 pint of water then add to 2 tsp of wood betony and infuse for ten minutes. Drink 2 cups daily until energy levels return to normal.

- Take up to 600 mg Korean ginseng for up to one month after lymphatic swellings subside.

Caution: Herbal remedies should only be used to support orthodox treatment; always consult a health-care professional in cases of glandular fever.

Seek professional help when

- **There is excessive thirst and frequent urination as this may suggest diabetes.**

- **Thyroid problems need professional treatment.**

- **Mumps affects adults.**

Hypoglycaemia sugar

Hypoglycaemia (low blood sugar) is caused by insulin overproduction. Glucose from the food we eat is converted into glycogen which is then stored in the liver and muscles. Glucose therefore needs to be regularly removed from the blood stream to ensure the right balance and high levels will trigger production of more insulin. There is evidence to suggest that too many refined sugars in the diet will overwork the pancreas, causing wide swings in blood sugar levels. Symptoms include constant hunger, dizziness, headaches, fatigue, irritability, memory lapses, visual disturbances, panic attacks and twitching limbs. Eating some sweet food usually brings rapid relief. Hypoglycaemia is a common syndrome with young, time-pressured adults who skip proper meals and can often be seen munching chocolate bars on the way home from work.

Treatment

- Take 1 or 2 drops of wormwood on the tongue to stimulate the digestion and help to normalize function.

- Drink infusions of chamomile, white horehound or wood betony instead of caffeine drinks during the day.

- Take two 200 mg of golden seal capsules or up to 600 mg of ginseng daily.

- Eat small, regular meals throughout the day and avoid alcohol, sugary snacks and refined carbohydrates.

- Chew liquorice root instead of sweets and chocolates.

Thyroid problems

Thyrotoxicosis (overactive thyroid)

The thyroid gland helps to control body metabolism and produces two important hormones which help our internal chemical factory to work normally and efficiently. In thyrotoxicosis (overactive thyroid) too much hormone is produced so the body goes into overdrive – everything speeds up and the result is weight loss, diarrhoea (*see page* 121), and sweating. Sufferers are often hyperactive – apparently full of energy and unable to sit still for very long. Bugleweed can be used specifically to reduce this overactivity.

Treatment

- Make an infusion containing two parts of bugleweed to one part each of motherwort and parsley. Drink a cup up to three times daily.

- Take 5 ml/1 tsp of valerian tincture in water three times daily or use two 200 mg capsules.

- Take supplements of vitamin A and C and calcium.

Myxedema

In myxedema (underactive thyroid), on the other hand, there is a shortage of important hormones: the result is a slow and sluggish metabolism, constipation (*see page* 120), weight gain, apathy and general lethargy. Sufferers have little energy and may appear mentally dull. The specific herb for an underactive thyroid is bladderwrack, which is a good source of iodine – a mineral that the thyroid uses to make its important hormones.

Treatment

- Make an infusion containing two parts bladderwrack to one part each of parsley, damiana, and wild oats. Drink a cup three times a day.

- Take supplements of ginseng and ginkgo.

- Take 5 ml/1 tsp each of wild oats and vervain tincture each morning if depression is a problem.

- Eat oatmeal porridge for breakfast.

- Avoid eating too much cabbage, cauliflower, spinach, Brussels sprouts, turnips, beans or soya products as these foods may deplete the thyroid still further.

- Take supplements of vitamin A, C, D, E, calcium, iodine and zinc.

Caution: Thyroid problems should always be referred to a health-care professional. Use self-help remedies to support treatment.

Mumps

Mumps (parotitis) is a viral disease which can affect a number of the body's glands: in children usually the salivary glands in the throat are affected, leading to difficulty swallowing, while in adults the infection may also lead to an inflammation of the testicles or ovaries and cause infertility. The pancreas can also be involved. For children the condition is usually mild and suitable for home treatment. Adult sufferers should seek professional help.

Treatment

- Make an antiseptic gargle by combining equal amounts of thyme and sage in an infusion and using a cup of the strained brew as a gargle and mouthwash. Repeat every 30–60 minutes while the symptoms are severe.

- Follow the recommendations for fevers given on page 127.

- Mix 50 ml/10 tsp of cleavers tincture, 25 ml/5 tsp of echinacea tincture and 25 ml/5 tsp of marigold tincture, and give in 5 ml/1 tsp doses three times daily before meals to counter infections and cleanse the system.

- Drink cups of skullcap, wood betony, or chamomile two or three times a day as a general relaxant.

Caution: Seek professional help in all cases.

Overcoming steroidal therapy

Synthetic steroids are a popular orthodox treatment for a number of inflammatory illnesses including arthritis (*see page* 131), skin disorders and asthma (*see page* 95). They can be very successful and bring rapid relief, but they do have side effects. Most notably, they tend to depress the body's own inflammatory response by the immune system; they affect white blood cells and reduce their ability to combat infections. Taking artificial corticosteroids also depresses the body's production of these chemicals, which are made in the adrenal glands, adjacent to the kidneys. Steroid-taking patients can thus become more susceptible to infections and often need a little gentle help when their treatment finishes to restore adrenal function. Borage is an excellent tonic for the adrenals.

Treatment

- Take 10 ml/2 tsp of fresh borage juice three times a day; alternatively, use 5 ml/1 tsp of tincture in a little water.

- Make an infusion containing equal parts gotu kola, borage and hawthorn, and drink a cup three times a day.

- Make a decoction containing two parts liquorice and wild yam root to one part ginger. Drink a glass three times a day.

- Take 600 mg of ginseng tablets daily.

- Take either echinacea or garlic capsules to boost the immune system.

Supplements and diet

- Bitter herbs will help to stimulate the system. Take a few drops of wormwood or dandelion root tincture on the tongue before meals. Bitter digestifs, popular in many parts of Europe, will have a similar effect.

- Avoid overloading the system with artificial chemicals – opt for organic produce and resist 'junk' foods. Take fewer artificial stimulants, including caffeine-containing drinks and alcohol.

- Eat small, regular meals rather than a single daily binge or constant 'grazing' on snack food.

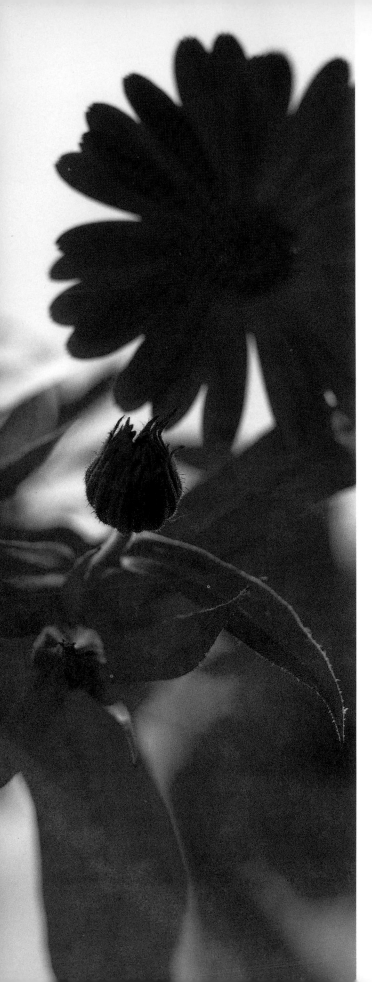

Skin and hair

Our skin forms a vital defensive barrier between us and the outside world: it allows cooling sweat to pass through, harbours a thriving community of bacteria to ward off unfriendly micro-organisms, and is home to a host of sensory organs. Its efficiency and quality are a good guide to our general health and wellbeing and we can all recognize when someone is 'glowing' with health. Herbal skin remedies usually focus on internal medication to restore a healthy balance.

Eczema

Eczema and dermatitis are both terms used to describe non-contagious inflammatory skin conditions. The skin is usually red and itching, with a rash or spots which can resemble small, 'weeping' blisters that ooze clear fluid, forming a crust. Allergic reaction is often to blame, with allergens ranging from nickel jewellery to food intolerance involving dairy products, wheat, eggs or fruits and vegetables (such as tomatoes, oranges, berry fruits, peppers and aubergines) that are rich in salicylates. Washing-up powder is another common culprit, as are house-dust mites and household pets. Anxiety and tension (*see page* 101) can also make the condition worse. In the elderly, poor circulation can lead to varicose eczema which may be associated with a tendency to develop varicose ulcers. Herbal treatment usually concentrates on cleansing and soothing internal remedies rather than on liberal use of external creams.

Treatment

- Make an infusion from equal amounts of red clover, heartsease, stinging nettle, skullcap and burdock leaves. Drink a cup three times a day. Add borage to the mixture to help strengthen the adrenal system if steroid creams have been used for any length of time.

- Evening primrose or borage (starflower) oil can help in some types of eczema – take 1000 mg in capsules daily.

- Use marigold or chamomile creams externally for dry eczema; try chickweed cream to help reduce itching.

- For weeping eczema make a wash by combining equal amounts of heartsease and marigold petals in a standard infusion, then strain and soak a compress in the mixture.

- Ensure an adequate supply of vitamins A, B, C and E in the diet, as well as magnesium, zinc and calcium – take supplements if necessary.

- Relieve itching with a lotion made from 25 ml/5 tsp each of borage juice, chickweed tincture, distilled witch hazel and rose water with 5 drops of rosemary oil.

Psoriasis

Psoriasis is a one of the most common skin complaints, affecting around one in a hundred people. It is characterized by itchy, dry skin covered with silvery scales that flake off to reveal inflamed, red areas. These patches can vary in size – from under 1 cm/$\frac{1}{2}$ in in diameter to covering almost the entire body in severe cases. Knees, legs, elbows, forearms and scalp are usually affected. The cause of psoriasis is complex and related to auto-immune disease and family tendency; in some cases there may be associated arthritis (*see page* 131). Anxiety and shocks (*see pages* 101, 103) can aggravate the condition.

Treatment

- Make a decoction of burdock, yellow dock and liquorice root and combine with an infusion of red clover and cleavers. Drink a cup three times a day.

- Take 600 mg of devil's claw root in tablets daily.

- Cleavers cream can be useful for small patches or in the early stages of psoriasis. Apply two or three times a day to affected areas.

- Psoriasis often seems to go with a tense, insular personality. Make an infusion of wood betony, skullcap and rose petals and drink a cup morning and night.

Seek professional help when

- **There are serious cuts or grazes which may require stitching.**

- **Burns are more than 2 cm/$\frac{4}{5}$ in in diameter (*see* Burns and scalds, *page* 146).**

- **A skin rash may be suspected shingles.**

- **There are changes to warts, freckles or moles, especially involving colour change or discharge.**

- **Allergic reactions involve major swelling and breathing difficulties.**

- **Sunburn is severe as this may be associated with heat stroke and dehydration.**

- If the scalp is affected use an infusion of rosemary, nettles and sage as a final rinse after shampooing.

- Take zinc, vitamin A, vitamin C and kelp tablets as supplements.

Acne

The characteristic pimples caused by inflamed sebaceous glands are all too familiar to teenagers. These glands open into hair follicles and produce an oily secretion known as sebum which helps to keep the skin soft, moist and supple. Excess oils can block skin pores and lead to bacterial infection, with pus-filled pimples, small cysts and blackheads. Typically, acne starts in the early teens and usually disappears by the mid-20s, although a tendency to spots can be a lifelong problem for some people.

Treatment
- Make a facial steamer by adding 1 tsp of dried lavender, yarrow and elder flowers to a basin of boiling water, and steam the face for 10–15 minutes.

- Make a lotion by mixing 10 ml/2 tsp of tea tree oil with 45 ml/3 tbsp each of distilled witch hazel and rose water.

- Take supplements of evening primrose oil, vitamin B, vitamin C and zinc.

- Blend three cabbage leaves with 50 ml/10 tsp of distilled witch hazel in a food processor and use as a lotion two times daily.

- Apply garlic cloves to pustules at night.

- If spots are worse before periods, women may find that taking chaste tree capsules can help. Alternatively, make a decoction of equal amounts of wild yam and *Dang Gui*, and drink 3 wine glass doses during the day.

- Cut down on the foods which might encourage sebaceous gland activity, such as refined carbohydrates (white sugar and flour), fried foods, animal fats, sweets and chocolates, alcohol and sweet, sugary drinks. Eat plenty of fresh vegetables and fruit.

Urticaria

These irritant weals which can suddenly appear on the skin are variously described as urticaria, hives or nettle rash. They usually fade within a few hours and are often associated with an allergic reaction to some substance – either something taken internally or with which there has been skin contact. Shellfish and strawberries are common culprits. Common garden plants can also cause hives, so take care with stinging nettles, hops, runner beans and borage.

Treatment
- Make an infusion containing equal amounts of agrimony, chamomile flowers, stinging nettles and heartsease. Drink a cup every two or three hours until the symptoms fade.

- Apply neat borage juice as a cooling lotion to ease irritation.

- Use chamomile cream on affected areas several times a day.

- An infusion of wood betony and skullcap night and morning can help if stress (*see page* 101) is a factor.

- Rub slices of onion or crushed cabbage leaves on to the affected area or use cabbage juice as a lotion.

Caution: In severe cases urticaria can be associated with swelling of the hands, face, arms, eyelids or throat and there may be painful joints or breathing problems which require emergency treatment.

Supplements and diet

- Diet is important for a healthy skin. Avoid refined carbohydrates, fatty and fried foods, dairy products and animal fats. Eat plenty of fresh fruits and vegetables, and drink at least 1½ litres/2¾ pints of water each day.

- Evening primrose and borage (starflower) oil are useful in numerous skin conditions. Take up to 1 gm a day; use capsules which also contain fish oils for psoriasis.

- Ensure an adequate intake of vitamin E, vitamin C and zinc. Pumpkin seeds and avocados are also useful sources.

Dandruff and seborrhoeic dermatitis

Dandruff is believed to be caused, in part, by a fungus (*Pityrosporum ovale*), although unlike similar infections it is not contagious. Wearing hats can make dandruff worse – the hot, damp environment so produced is ideal for encouraging fungal growth. Using medicated shampoos can exacerbate the condition because they contain detergents which can impede scalp secretions and natural bacteria.

Treatment

- Make a herbal shampoo by mixing 2 tbsp of soft soap with a cup of methyl alcohol and 2 tsp each of fresh rosemary leaves and washed stinging nettle root. Leave to infuse for two weeks, then strain and use as ordinary shampoo.

- Use an infusion of rosemary, marigold, sage, or stinging nettle or a decoction of burdock root as a final rinse after shampooing.

- Rub live yoghurt into the scalp after washing; leave for 15 minutes and then rinse well.

Alopecia

Hair loss and baldness in ageing men tends to be hereditary and non-reversible. Where hair loss is sudden or patchy as in alopecia, or stress (*see page* 101), vitamin deficiency may be to blame. It is most common in teenagers and young adults.

Treatment

- Apply arnica cream to bald patches but do not use on unbroken skin.

- Take vitamin B complex, zinc and evening primrose or borage (starflower) oil supplements.

- Use infusions of rosemary, sage, or stinging nettle as a final hair rinse. If possible use stinging nettle root in a decoction rather than as an infusion of the herb.

- To combat stress, make an infusion of skullcap and wood betony tea and drink 3 cups a day; take 600 mg of Siberian ginseng daily.

Athlete's foot and ringworm

Athlete's foot and ringworm are fungal infections which are caused by various *Tinea* spp. and affect different parts of the body. Athlete's foot occurs in the space between the toes and toenails, *Tinea favosa* affects the nails, and other varieties occur on the body, scalp, groin and beard area. Depending on the infecting fungus, there may be inflammation and itching or simply scaling of the skin and general discomfort. Like all their species, the yeasts causing athlete's foot and ringworm thrive in warm, damp places, so good, sensible hygiene – making sure that the toes and groin are well dried after bathing, that hats are not too tight, and that shoes are comfortable – is important. Using creams based on antifungal herbs can help.

Treatment

- Apply a little tea tree, echinacea, or marigold cream to the affected area night and morning.

- Use the fresh sap from an aloe vera leaf on the affected area night and morning.

- Take 600 mg echinacea, 600 mg golden seal and 2 gm garlic daily in capsules to boost the immune system and combat infection.

- Use a nightly foot bath containing 10 drops of myrrh tincture or 5 drops of tea tree oil.

- If the scalp is affected use a strained marigold infusion as a rinse or add 5 drops of tea tree or thyme oil to the rinsing water after shampooing.

- Take 10 ml/2 tsp fresh cleavers juice three times a day.

- Make an infusion containing equal amounts of cleavers, chickweed and gotu kola, and drink a cup three times daily.

Verrucas and warts

Warts are benign lumps in the skin caused by a virus which makes the cells multiply abnormally quickly. They are usually found on the hands, knees and face, and are mildly contagious but usually quite harmless; most will disappear of their own accord – eventually. Verrucas are warts that occur on the soles of the feet. Because they are always being walked on, the small growths can become painful and are often covered by thickened areas of skin or calluses. Ring plasters and callous pads can provide some relief.

Treatment
- The fresh sap from dandelion stems or greater celandine (*Chelidonium major*) applied to the wart night and morning is usually effective.

- Use 1–2 drops of neat tea tree oil night and morning.

- Use a little powdered slippery elm mixed with water as a paste and apply night and morning with a small plaster to keep the mix in place.

- Take two 200 mg of echinacea twice a day to boost the immune system.

Caution: Professional help is needed for warts which appear to erupt on the site of moles or which start to bleed or change colour.

Bruises

Bruises are caused by blood escaping from damaged underlying blood vessels following injury. A tendency to bruise may be related to problems with the blood's clotting ability or it could simply suggest that small blood vessels are comparatively thin and easily damaged, as is often the case in otherwise fit and healthy women.

Treatment
- Apply arnica or comfrey creams if the skin is unbroken. If the skin is broken use marigold cream instead.

- Soak a compress in a hot infusion of arnica, comfrey, chickweed, hyssop, hemp agrimony, fenugreek or St John's wort.

- Use mashed cabbage leaves as a poultice.

- The common garden daisy (*Bellis perennis*) was once known as bruisewort and was a popular folk remedy for all sorts of bruising.

- Take homeopathic Arnica 6x or Bach Flower Rescue Remedy (*see page* 105) internally to calm the sufferer and encourage more rapid healing.

- An ice pack of frozen peas provides ideal emergency treatment to relieve the pain of a new bruise. Alternate that with a hot water bottle to encourage reabsorption of blood and bring more rapid relief.

Burns and scalds

Scalds are caused by moist heat and burns by dry heat. Burns are potential medical emergencies and only the most minor should be treated at home.

Treatment
- For less severe injuries, run cold water over the affected area or use an ice pack of frozen peas to cool it down and ease the immediate pain. Keeping the injury cool for two or three hours can often help significantly.

- After cooling the area, use fresh sap from an aloe vera leaf directly on the affected area, or apply a little St John's wort or marigold infused oil.

- Drink an infusion of stinging nettle, St John's wort and vervain tea to combat shock.

- Raw grated potato can be used as a poultice.

Caution: Burns are classified in six degrees: anything above second degree (redness, soreness and blistering) should be treated in hospital. Any burn more than about 5 cm/2 in across, or greater in severity than first degree, should be seen by a doctor as soon as possible. Second degree burns or above may be accompanied by shock.

Cuts and grazes

There are many herbal alternatives to orthodox antiseptic creams: you can bathe wounds using herbal infusions as a wash and then apply suitable herbal creams or infused oils as necessary.

Treatment

- Always bathe cuts and grazes before applying creams: either rinse the wound under running water or use cotton wool soaked in a strained infusion of marigold or St John's wort taking care to wipe from the centre to the edge of the graze to clear any grime. Press a clean tissue or gauze pad over the injury for a few minutes to stop bleeding.

- Apply a little marigold, echinacea, chickweed, St John's wort or tea tree creams.

- As an alternative, use fresh aloe vera sap or aloe vera cream.

- Bruised shepherd's purse, hyssop, bistort, self-heal, or yarrow leaves can all be used as poultices or as emergency first aid in the countryside.

Sunburn

Ozone depletion in the atmosphere is allowing more damaging ultraviolet rays to reach the earth's surface, so it makes sense to wear large-brimmed hats, protective sun-glasses and long-sleeved shirts. Protective sun-block creams are essential, but if you do get burned, herbal remedies can help.

Treatment

- Pack a bottle containing 25 ml/5 tsp of infused St John's wort oil with 25 drops of lavender oil when holidaying in hot climates. Apply liberally to damaged, sunburned skin.

- Fresh aloe vera sap or aloe vera creams can also be effective.

- Drink an infusion of elder flower, yarrow and boneset to encourage sweating and cool the skin.

- Bathe the skin in a cooled infusion of marigold petals and common plantain leaves.

- Take supplements of beta carotene, vitamins A and C and zinc to combat skin damage.

Insect bites and stings

For most people insect bites and stings cause little more than a local irritation which eases in a few days. For an unfortunate minority stings can lead to severe allergic reactions which can be fatal. Immediate emergency medical treatment is vital in such cases.

Treatment

- Use creams containing St John's wort, marigold, sage or lemon balm to ease irritation. Infusions of any of these herbs can be used as a wash to bathe the weeping sores which develop from some types of insect bites in sensitive individuals.

- Use the fresh sap from an aloe vera leaf or apply aloe vera ointment.

- A slice of fresh raw onion will ease bee and wasp stings.

- Fresh plantain or lemon balm leaves rubbed onto the bite or sting will bring relief.

- If bites become infected, echinacea or tea tree cream can be helpful.

- Tea tree, lemon balm, and citronella oils diluted in almond oil and used as a rub on exposed skin can all help to keep insects at bay. Burn citronella candles at barbecues or spray some of these oils, well-diluted in water, over clothing.

Caution: If pain and swelling do not respond to treatment or if the sufferer feels faint or unwell, seek medical help. With allergy to stings, there is a danger of anaphylactic shock. Emergency treatment with an injection of adrenaline and antihistamine may need to be administered.

Splinters

Use a little chickweed, marshmallow, or slippery elm ointment to help draw stubborn splinters: apply, cover with a small bandage, and leave for a few hours before extracting the splinter with tweezers or a clean needle.

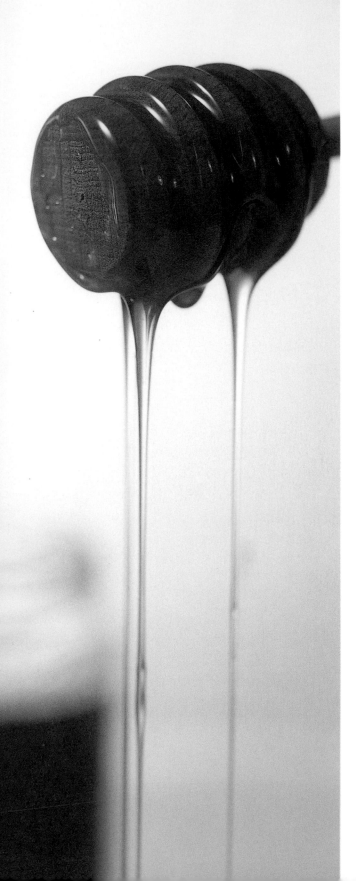

Babies and children

In general, children's ailments are self-limiting and mild, although sometimes symptoms can be dramatic, with sudden fevers and soaring temperatures. Children's metabolism is much faster than that of adults, with a rapid pulse rate and quicker breathing rate, and illness can appear to develop more rapidly as well. Herbs can provide a gentle remedy for even quite young babies; older children may need some persuasion or liberal use of sweetening honey to make some remedies more palatable (children under the age of 2 should not be given unpasteurized honey).

Colic

The spasms and discomfort of colic can often be caused by problems at feeding times: rushing feeds or tension transferred from mother to baby inevitably causes upsets. Check the baby's diet (or your own if breastfeeding) for likely irritants such as hot spices, cow's milk or wheat, and ensure that both mother and baby are relaxed and calm at mealtimes.

Treatment

- Make an infusion containing equal amounts of catmint and dill, and give 5–15 ml/1–3 tsp diluted with water up to four times a day. Small babies will often happily drink herbal infusions if they have been introduced early enough.

- Homeopathic chamomile (Chamomilla 3x) can be given in drop doses every 15 minutes to relieve colic.

- To calm breastfeeding mothers, drink a standard infusion of skullcap, vervain, wood betony or chamomile tea before feeds.

- Make an infusion from 15 g/¹⁄₂ oz of chamomile flowers and ¹⁄₂ litre/1 pint of water. Use it to soak a compress and apply to the baby's abdomen to relieve colicky pains.

Gastric upsets

Childhood diarrhoea and biliousness are common in immature digestive systems. They can be related to migraines in later life, and thus may be linked to food intolerance. Always ensure adequate fluid intake as children easily become dehydrated.

Treatment

- Agrimony infusion is ideal for children. Use ¹⁄₂ to 1 cup as a simple remedy for diarrhoea or combine with an equal amount of wood betony if the upset is associated with headaches and nausea.

Caution: Always seek professional advice for children's gastric upsets which last for more than 12 hours.

Nappy rash

The painful irritation of nappy rash can be caused by irregular or inefficient nappy changes and cleansing, but it can also be related to digestive problems and yeast infections. Nappy rash is a common and distressing problem. If breastfeeding, reduce your intake of foods likely to encourage fungal growths, such as refined carbohydrates, junk foods, preserved or salted foods and milk products.

Treatment

- Add 10 drops of tea tree to 10 ml/2 tsp of infused comfrey oil. Apply a little of the oil to the affected area at each nappy change, making sure that the baby is well dried. Use a cool hair dryer if necessary and leave the nappy off for as long as possible.

- Use an infusion of heartsease as a soothing wash for the affected area before applying the above comfrey oil mixture.

- Proprietary comfrey or marigold ointments can be used instead of the home-made mixture.

Seek professional help when

- **There is severe diarrhoea or vomiting, or milder diarrhoea which continues for more than 12 hours.**

- **Temperatures are above 39°C/102.2°F for more than a couple of hours.**

- **There are convulsions, breathing problems, or unusual drowsiness.**

- **There is an unusual, high-pitched cry.**

Cradle cap

Cradle cap is a scaly dermatitis which can affect the scalps of small babies and can be due to overactive sweat glands. It is not serious or contagious although mothers tend to find it unsightly.

Treatment
- Combine infused oils of heartsease and marigold and massage a little into the baby's scalp several times day. Be especially careful with newborn babies whose fontanelles (soft spots in the skull) may not have closed completely.

- Use a heartsease infusion to bathe the baby's head at bath time.

Sleeplessness

Sleepless babies soon become a problem for the entire family, leading to irritability and tensions in relationships. The cause may be nothing more complex than a hot room, colic (*see page* 149) or hunger, so ensure that the baby is comfortable and feels safe and secure. If sleeplessness continues to the toddler stage, give lots of cuddles and reassurance – and relaxing herbs to the entire household.

Treatment
- Add 1 cup of chamomile infusion or 2 drops of chamomile oil to bath water each night. Agitate the water well to ensure good dispersion before bathing the baby.

- Gentle massage can help calm small babies: stroke forearms slowly in one direction repeatedly rather than trying body massage. Apply a little very dilute mix (1 drop of chamomile oil in 20 ml/4 tsp sweet almond oil) before massaging.

- Give an infusion (10 g/$\frac{1}{3}$ oz to $\frac{1}{2}$ litre/1 pint of water) at night using chamomile flowers, Californian poppy, or lemon balm. Flavour with honey or lemon juice as required.

- Ensure that the diet is adequate, with a good vitamin and mineral intake. Avoid caffeine if breastfeeding and check foods for artificial colourants or additives if the child is taking solids.

Teething

Teething usually starts from around four months, although in some cases it can be a problem from a few weeks after birth. The result is often sleepless nights and tension for the entire family.

Treatment
- Mix 2 drops each of chamomile, sage and rosemary oils in 5 ml/1 tsp of almond oil, smear a small amount of the oil on to your finger, and gently rub the baby's gums with it. Repeat three or four times a day as necessary.

- Give sedative herbs like lime flowers or chamomile in weak infusions (25–50 ml/5–10 tsp) before feeds.

- Use homeopathic Chamomilla 3x pillules or drops as required.

Measles

A highly contagious viral disease, measles is characterized by the typical symptoms of a heavy cold, with a harsh dry cough, a blotchy rash usually starting behind the ears and bloodshot, light-sensitive eyes. It usually occurs in local epidemics, and complications include pneumonia and middle ear infections.

Treatment
- Make an infusion from equal amounts of hyssop, marshmallow leaf and ribwort plantain, and give a half a cup up to four times daily. Use smaller doses for younger children.

- Give one 200 mg echinacea capsule or 20 drops to 5 ml/1 tsp of echinacea tincture three times daily before meals. If children cannot swallow capsules or tablets, then open the capsule and mix the powdered contents with a 1 tsp of honey.

- Use eyebright or self-heal infusions, well strained in eyebaths (*see* Useful eyebaths, *page* 136) to soothe irritation.

- Sponge feverish children with a marigold or basil infusion as necessary.

Caution: Always seek professional help for measles.

Chickenpox

In children, chickenpox is usually a mild, if highly contagious, infection. It is characterized by rashes which soon turn into spots, and then blister and lead to scabs. Spots are most common on the scalp, face and body and are very irritating. Scratching or damaging the scabs can lead to scars, so take great care when bathing infected children. There is often a mild fever (*see page* 127). In adults the same virus produces shingles (*see page* 129) which can be severe and lead to lingering nerve pain.

Treatment

- Make a lotion from equal amounts of chickweed infusion, borage juice and distilled witch hazel. Apply to irritant skin rashes every one to two hours or as required.

- Give the child two 200 mg of echinacea capsules or 5 ml/ 1 tsp of echinacea tincture three times daily before meals.

- As a general relaxant, give the child a skullcap, wood betony, or chamomile infusion two to three times daily.

- Gently sponge feverish children with a cooled marigold, borage, or basil infusion.

Nits and head lice

Lice and their eggs (nits) are increasingly common in school outbreaks and are easily spread. Suspect infection if children persistently scratch their heads.

Treatment

- Mix together equal amounts of tea tree, thyme and lemon essential oils, or use them separately if more convenient. Add 10 drops to ½ litre/1 pint of warm water and use as a final hair rinse after shampooing. Repeat each day until the infection clears.

- Alternatively, add the same selection of oils to 10 ml/2 tsp of sweet almond oil and soak a fine-toothed comb in the mixture before combing the child's hair very thoroughly. Repeat twice a day until the infection clears.

Worms

Threadworms and pinworms can be common in children; they are highly contagious and easily spread to the entire family, including adult members. Good domestic hygiene is needed if the rest of the household is to avoid infection. Female worms lay their eggs at the anus at night, so examine the child's bottom before bedtime and remove the worms where possible. Treatment needs to be repeated at fortnightly intervals to mirror the worm's life cycle.

Treatment

- Add 10 drops each of wormwood and fennel tincture to a glass of carrot juice. Stir well and give every morning before breakfast for four days. Repeat the treatment two weeks later.

- Garlic also clears worms. Give 1–4 garlic capsules each morning, or finely chop a clove and mix it with a little honey stirred into a cup of warm milk.

- Cabbage is another effective remedy. Juice fresh leaves in a food processor or juicer and use 60 ml/4 tbsp as an alternative to the carrot juice.

Bed-wetting

Regular bed-wetting in young children can be associated with minor urinary infections, dietary imbalance, physical problems with the urinary tract or emotional upsets. Identifying the cause is important and medical investigation is obviously needed if there is a physical reason for the disorder.

Treatment

- Make an infusion from equal amounts of cornsilk and St John's wort, and give 30–45 ml/2–3 tbsp with a little honey three times a day.

- Combine equal amounts of horsetail, shepherd's purse and mullein tincture, and give 20–60 drops (depending on age) three times daily.

Hyperactivity

All children are active, but when they become hyperactive the whole family can suffer: typical problems can include sleeplessness, poor attention span, frequent tears and aggressive behaviour. Food intolerance or pollution are often to blame or there may be emotional difficulties.

Treatment

- Make an infusion containing equal amounts of wood betony, self-heal and borage. Give ½ to 1 cup up to three times a day.

- Check that the diet contains an adequate supply of B vitamins and minerals like zinc and iron.

- Avoid all artificial colourings, preservatives and other additives, and strictly control the intake of sugar, chocolate, milk and caffeine.

- Evening primrose or borage (starflower) oil as a dietary supplement can help – give 250–500 mg daily. Zinc supplements can also be useful.

- Try to introduce deep breathing exercises on a daily basis to encourage relaxation.

- If environmental pollution is contributing to the problem, give kelp supplements which can help cleanse heavy metals from the system.

Travel sickness

Nausea and vomiting caused by travelling is often related to lack of air, diesel fumes and restricted vision, which upsets the balance of the inner ear. It is especially common in children whose ears have increased sensitivity. Make sure the car windows are open and try to spend as much time above deck as possible on sea journeys.

Treatment

- Ginger in any form is ideal: take capsules, drops of dilute tincture, ginger wine, teas or, for younger children, crystallized ginger sweets, ginger ale, or ginger biscuits 20–30 minutes before travelling. Repeat as required. Galangal acts similarly to ginger.

- Give the child a cup of chamomile, lemon balm or meadowsweet infusion before travelling, or use 2–3 drops of tincture on the tongue at regular intervals during the journey.

Doses for children and the elderly

Doses for children and the very elderly need to be reduced depending on age, body weight, and metabolism. For children use the following proportions:

Age	Dose
0–1 year	5 per cent of adult dose
1–2 years	10 per cent of adult dose
3–4 years	20 per cent of adult dose
5–6 years	30 per cent of adult dose
7–8 years	40 per cent of adult dose
9–10 years	50 per cent of adult dose
11–12 years	60 per cent of adult dose
	80 per cent of adult dose
	100 per cent of adult dose

For those over 70 give 80 per cent of the adult dose, for those over 80 give 70 per cent of the adult dose, and for over-90s give 60 per cent of the adult dose.

These guidelines are of necessity approximate – much will depend on individual vitality.

Directory of common names

Common name	Botanical name	Common name	Botanical name	Common name	Botanical name
Agrimony	*Agrimonia eupatoria*	Dill	*Anethum graveolens*	Melilot	*Melitotus officinale*
Aloe	*Aloe vera*	Echinacea (Purple		Milk thistle	*Silybum marianum*
Arnica	*Arnica montana*	coneflower)	*Echinacea spp (E. purpurea,*	Milk vetch	
Basil	*Ocimum basilicum*		*E. angustifolia, E. pallida)*	(Huang Qi)	*Astragalus membranaceous*
Bilberry	*Vaccinium myrtillus*	Elder	*Sambucus nigra*	Motherwort	*Leonurus cardiaca*
Bistort	*Polygonum bistorta*	Elecampane	*Inula helenium*	Mullein	*Verbascum thapsus*
Black cohosh	*Cimicifuga racemosa*	Eucalyptus	*Eucalyptus globulus*	Myrrh	*Commiphora myrrha*
Black haw	*Virburnum prunifolium*	Evening primrose	*Oenetheris biennis*	Nutmeg	*Myristica fragrans*
Bladderwrack	*Fucus vesiculosis*	Eyebright	*Euphrasia officinalis*	Parsley	*Petroselinum crispum*
Blue cohosh	*Caulophyllum thalictroides*	Fennel	*Foeniculum vulgare*	Passion flower	*Passiflora incarnata*
Boneset	*Eupatorium perfoliatum*	Fenugreek	*Trigonella foenum-graecum*	Peppermint	*Mentha X piperita*
Borage	*Borago officinalis*	Feverfew	*Tanacetum parthenium*	Raspberry	*Rubus idaeus*
Buchu	*Agathosma betulina*	Flowery knotweed		Red clover	*Trifolium pratense*
Buckwheat	*Fagopyrum esculentum*	(He Shou Wu)	*Polygonum multiflorum*	Reishi	*Ganoderma lucidem*
Bugleweed	*Lycopus virginicus*	Forsythia		Ribwort plantain	*Plantago lanceolata*
Burdock	*Arctium lappa*	(Lian Qiao)	*Forsythia suspensa*	Rose	*Rosa* spp
Californian poppy	*Eschscholtzia californica*	Fringe tree	*Chionanthus virginianum*	Rosemary	*Rosmarinus officinalis*
Catmint	*Nepeta cataria*	Galangal	*Alpina officinarum*	Sage	*Salvia officinalis*
Cayenne	*Capsicum frutescens*	Garlic	*Allium sativa*	St John's wort	*Hypericum perforatum*
Celery	*Apium graveolens*	Ginger	*Zingiber officinale*	Sandalwood	*Santalum alba*
Chamomile	*Matricaria recutita*	Ginkgo	*Ginkgo biloba*	Saw palmetto	*Serenoa repens*
Chaste tree	*Vitex agnus-castus*	Ginseng	*Panax ginseng*	Self-heal	
Chickweed	*Stellaria media*	Goat's rue	*Galega officinalis*	(Hu Ku Cao)	*Prunella vulgaris*
Chinese angelica		Golden rod	*Solidago vigaurea*	Shepherd's purse	*Capsella bursa-pastoris*
(Dang Gui)	*Angelica polymorpha*	Golden seal	*Hydrastis canadensis*	Siberian ginseng	*Eleutherococcus senticosus*
	var. *sinesis*	Gotu kola	*Centella asiatica*	Silverweed	*Potentilla anserina*
Chinese rhubarb		Ground ivy	*Glechoma hederacea*	Skullcap	*Scutellaria lateriflora*
(Da Huang)	*Rheum palmatum*	Hawthorn	*Crataegus laevigata;*	Slippery elm	*Ulmus rubra*
Chrysanthemum			*C. monogyna*	Stinging nettle	*Urtica dioica*
(Ju Hua)	*Dendranthema X*	Heartsease	*Viola tricolor*	Tea tree	*Melaleuca alternifolia*
	grandiflorum	Hemp agrimony	*Eupatorium cannabium*	Thyme	*Thymus vulgaris*
Cleavers	*Galium aparine*	Helonias	*Chamaelirium luteum*	Valerian	*Valeriana officinalis*
Cloves	*Syzygium aromaticum*	Hops	*Humulus lupulus*	Vervain	*Verbena officinalis*
Comfrey	*Symphytum officinalis*	Horsetail	*Equisetum arvense*	White deadnettle	*Lamium album*
Common plantain	*Plantago major*	Hyssop	*Hyssopus officinale*	White horehound	*Marrubium vulgare*
Cornflower	*Centaurea cyanus*	Ispagula	*Plantago psyllium; P. ovata*	Wild oats	*Avena sativa*
Cornsilk	*Zea mays*	Lady's mantle	*Alchemilla xanthoclora*	White willow	*Salix alba*
Cowslip	*Primula veris*	Lavender	*Lavendula angustifolia*	Wild yam	*Dioscorea villosa*
Cramp bark	*Viburnum opulus*	Lemon	*Citrus lemon*	Winter cherry	
Cranberry	*Vaccinium macrocarpon*	Lemon balm	*Melissa officinalis*	(Ashwagandha)	*Withania somnifera*
Damiana	*Turnera dIffusa* var.	Lime	*Tilia cordata*	Witch hazel	*Hamamelis virginiana*
	aphrodisiaca	Liquorice	*Glycyrrhiza glabra*	Wood betony	*Stachys officinalis*
Dandelion	*Taraxacum officinale*	Marigold	*Calendula officinalis*	Wormwood	*Artemisia absinthum*
Devil's claw	*Harpagophytum*	Marshmallow	*Althaea officinale*	Yarrow	*Achillea millefolium*
	procumbens	Meadowsweet	*Filipendula ulmaria*	Yellow dock	*Rumex crispus*

Glossary

Adrenal cortex part of the adrenal gland located above the kidneys, which produces several steroidal hormones.

Adrenal stimulant a stimulant for the adrenal glands.

Agni a concept in Ayurvedic medicine sometimes described as 'digestive fire'; it is central to good health and ensures absorption of nutrients from food and destruction of pathogens (disease producing organisms).

Allopathic prevalent system of Western medicine which treats illness by prescribing substances to provoke an opposite condition from the disease - thus a fever is treated with temperature suppressants or an ache with painkillers.

Analgesic relieves pain.

Anaphrodisiac reduces sexual desire and excitement.

Anodyne allays pain.

Anthelmintic substances which destroy parasitic worms or expel them from the body.

Antiallergenic relieves allergic symptoms caused by a hypersensitive response to a foreign protein.

Antibacterial destroys or inhibits the growth of bacteria.

Antibiotic destroys or inhibits the growth of micro-organisms such as bacteria and fungi.

Anticatarrhal reduces the production of mucus.

Anticoagulant substances which prevent clotting or clumping of platelets (microscopic coagulants found in blood) to form blood clots.

Antidiarrhoeal substances which stop diarrhoea or soothe bowel irritation.

Antieczema substances which relieve the symptoms of eczema.

Antiemetic counters vomiting (emesis) and nausea.

Antifungal destroys or inhibits the growth of fungi.

Antihidrotic reduces sweating.

Antihistamine substances that prevent production of histamine (a compound produced in the body to combat inflammation) which is also associated with allergic response.

Antiinflammatory reduces inflammation.

Antimicrobial destroys or inhibits the growth of micro-organisms such as bacteria and fungi.

Antioxidant prevents or slows the natural deterioration of cells that occurs as they age due to oxidation.

Antiparasitic combats parasites as in anthelmintics *q.v.*

Antipruritic relieves intense itching.

Antipyretic reduces fevers as in febrifuge *q.v.*

Antirheumatic relieves the symptoms of rheumatism.

Antiscorbutic counters the symptoms of scurvy, a vitamin C deficiency disorder.

Antiseptic controls or prevents infection.

Antispasmodic reduces muscle spasm and tension.

Antithrombotic counters the production of blood clots.

Antitussive inhibits the cough reflex, helping to stop coughing.

Antiviral destroys or inhibits the growth of viruses.

Astringent used to describe a herb which will precipitate proteins from the surface of cells or membranes causing tissues to contract and tighten; forms a protective coating and stops bleeding and discharges.

Bergapten a chemical in the furano-coumarin *q.v.* group found in a number of herbs, including celery seed.

Bile stimulant thick, bitter fluid secreted by the liver and stored in the gall bladder which aids the digestion of fats.

Bitter stimulates secretion of digestive juices.

Bitter digestive herb a bitter herb which stimulates the digestive system.

Caprylic acid a fatty acid found in breast milk, currently used in the treatment of candidiasis.

Cardiotonic heart tonic.

Carminative expels gas from the stomach and intestines to relieve flatulence, digestive colic and gastric discomfort.

Cell proliferator encourages cell growth.

Centaurine a bitter tasting plant constituent.

Circulatory stimulant increases blood flow.

Coumarins active plant constituent which affects blood clotting.

Decoction a water-based herbal extract made by simmering the plant material in water.

Demulcent softens and soothes damaged or inflamed surfaces, such as the gastric mucous membranes.

Dermatitis skin inflammation.

Diaphoretic increases sweating.

Diuretic encourages urine flow.

Emollient softens and soothes the skin.

Ephedrine an alkaloid (type of chemical) found in a number of plants, notable *Ephedra* spp. used in the relief of asthma and hay fever.

Expectorant enhances the secretion or sputum from the respiratory tract so that it is easier to cough up.

Febrifuge reduces fever.

Flavonoids active plant constituents which improve the circulation and may also have diuretic, anti-inflammatory and antispasmodic effects.

Haemostatic stops bleeding.

Heilpraktiker a German medical qualification for alternative practitioners which has equivalent status to orthodox medical training.

Hepatic restorative restorative remedy for liver function.

Hepatic tonic liver tonic.

Hypertension high blood pressure.

Hypertensive raises blood pressure.

Hypnotic a substance that encourages sleep by depressing brain function.

Hypoglycaemic reduces blood sugar levels.

Hypolipidaemic reduces lipid (fats, steroids etc.) levels.

Hypotensive lowers blood pressure.

Immune stimulant stimulates the immune system.

Infusion a water-based herbal extract made by immersing the plant material in boiling water.

Laxative encourages bowel motions.

Lymphatic cleanser a substance which will cleanse the lymphatic system.

Lymphatic tonic tonic for the lymphatic system.

Menstrual regulator regulates the menstrual cycle.

Mucilaginous a substances containing mucilage – complex sugar molecules found in plants that are soft and slippery and provide protection for the mucous membranes and inflamed surfaces.

Mycoprotein protein derived from mould and fungi.

Nervine herb that affects the nervous system and which may be stimulating or sedating.

Nutritive substances providing nutrition.

Oestrogenic related to, or having a similar action to, the female hormone oestrogen.

Peripheral vasodilator relaxes (dilates) surface blood vessels, encouraging the blood circulation.

Photosensitivity sensitive to light.

Phytotherapists a French term for medical herbalists which is becoming more widespread across Europe.

Poultice powders, dried or fresh herbs mixed with hot water and applied to the skin to treat a wide range of ailments.

Prana the body's vital energy as defined in Ayurvedic medicine; often equated with breath.

Qi (ch'i) the body's vital energy as defined in Chinese medicine.

Rhizome a thick horizontal plant stem partly along and partly under ground sending out shoots above and roots below.

Rubefacient a substance which stimulates blood flow to the skin causing local reddening.

Rutin a type of flavonoid found in plants such as buckwheat and believed to strengthen blood vessels.

Salicylates a group of chemicals found in numerous plants which are generally anti-inflammatory; the drug aspirin is a type of salicylate.

Saponins active plant constituents similar to soap and producing a lather with water. They can irritate the mucous membranes of the digestive tract which, by reflex, has an expectorant action. Some saponins are chemically similar to steroidal hormones.

Sedative reduces anxiety and tension.

Stimulant increases activity.

Styptic stops external bleeding.

Testosterogenic related to, or having a similar action to, the male hormone testosterone.

Thujone a plant constituent found in such herbs as wormwood which stimulates the brain; it can be toxic in large quantities and should be avoided by epileptics as it may trigger attacks.

Tincture liquid herbal extract made by soaking plant material in a mixture of alcohol and water.

Tonify/tonifying a tonic action: strengthening and restoring for the system.

Uterine stimulant stimulates the womb.

Vasoconstrictor tenses or constricts blood vessels.

Index

Page numbers in italic
refer to the illustrations.

Acknowledgements

The author wishes to thank her herbal colleagues and patients who have provided so many insights into the value of our healing herbs over so many years. Thanks are also due to JEC and MHO for their support and patience during the writing of this book.

The publishers would like to thank the following people and organizations for their invaluable help with props and locations for the photography in this book:

Richard Adams and **Michelle Wosner**, **The Archway Clinic of Herbal Medicine**, Archway, London

Dr Susanna Jiang, **Jiang Clinic/Herbal Inn**, Finchley, London

Neal's Yard Remedies, Covent Garden, London

Ginkgo Garden Centre, Ravenscourt Park, London

All photographs appearing in this book were taken by Colin Bowling for Octopus Publishing Group, except for the following:

AKG, London / Erich Lessing 10 / Erich Lessing/Bibliotheque Nationale, Paris 13 / Erich Lessing/Oesterreichische Nationalbibliothek, Vienna 11 / Uffizi, Florence 14
Bridgeman Art Library / National Palace Museum, Taipei, Taiwan 18
Corbis UK Ltd / Bettmann 12 / Historical Picture Archive 21, E.T. Archive 15, 16
Octopus Publishing Group Ltd / W.F. Davidson 41 *top left*. From 'The Golden Mirror' 19 *bottom right* / From 'Ling Shu Su Wen Chieh Yao' 20 / Seibi Wake 19 *top left*

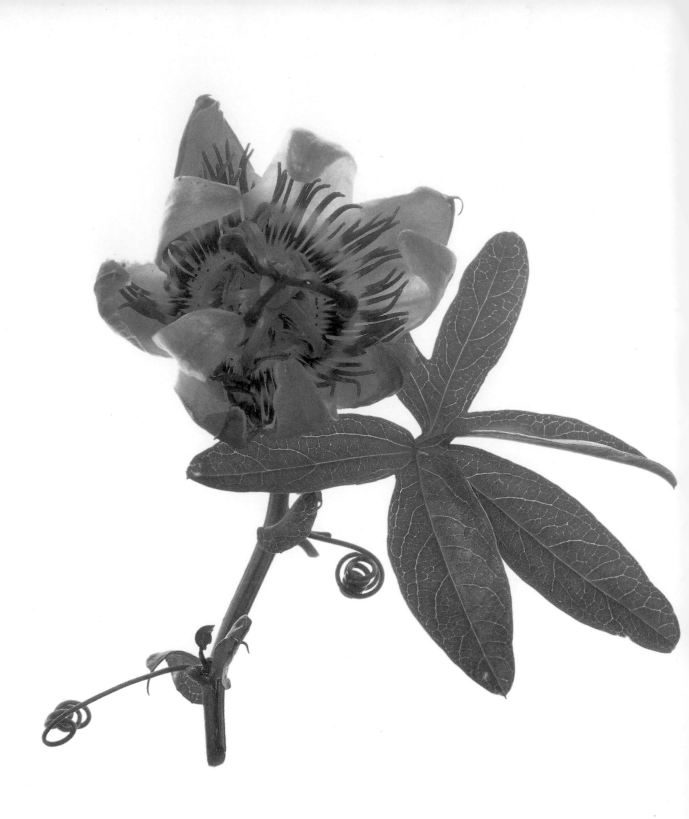

Passion flower *Passiflora incarnata*